Your Stomach Is A Liar !

Your Stomach Is A Liar !

Basic Nutrition, Weight Control and Misinterpreting Hunger

Edward Goodrich, M.D., F.A.C.S.

iUniverse, Inc.

New York Lincoln Shanghai

Your Stomach Is A Liar !
Basic Nutrition, Weight Control and Misinterpreting Hunger

iUniverse books may be ordered through booksellers or by contacting:

iUniverse
2021 Pine Lake Road, Suite 100
Lincoln, NE 68512
www.iuniverse.com
1-800-Authors (1-800-288-4677)

ISBN-13: 978-0-595-40407-0 (pbk)
ISBN-13: 978-0-595-84782-2 (ebk)
ISBN-10: 0-595-40407-3 (pbk)
ISBN-10: 0-595-84782-X (ebk)

Printed in the United States of America

To All My Children

and

Their's Forever

Author's Preface and Acknowledgment

This book is a result of numerous frustrating conversations held with obese patients over a period of many years. Whether the cause of obesity alluded to in the book's title is a significant source of this country's widespread problem, leading to consequent overindulgence, remains to be seen. To counter possible misunder standing, I have tried to present reliable, yet simplified, nutritional information on what is a remarkably complex subject. The success of this attempt will be impossible to measure and, although I have received much help in the writing, errors are uniquely mine. I wish the weight afflicted success in their attempt to understand and to learn to control their hunger, and I hope the information presented here helps the weight burdened to lose.

If any errors have survived rigorous proofing by my son and friends, especially Alfred, Hillary and Carl, they belong entirely to me. I would appreciate having them brought to my attention at the website: www.stomachliar.com. I am particularly indebted to my friend, Milt Overall, for his stimulative spurring. Should any part of this book be obscure, I will be happy to try to elaborate where necessary or helpful. Naturally, anyone seriously seeking to lose from a few to many pounds should consult their own health care provider.

E. O. Goodrich, M.D,. F.A.C.S.
Ardmore, PA
June 2006

Contents

Part Three: Your Stomach, The Liar

List of Figures and Tables

Introductory Chapter: Philosophy behind this book and the Author's hopes for usefulness to the reader

Introduction

"But Doctor, I don't eat that much" has been said to me repeatedly throughout my long medical career, usually by people who could be classified as obese, sometimes seriously or even morbidly so. For many years I accepted that statement as evidence of denial on the part of the speaker and that he or she lacked adequate insight into the true source of their obesity with which they might be better able to control the problem. However, the obvious sincerity of each speaker motivated me to try to understand, better, the reason for this common, almost universal, claim.

Over many years in Surgical, then General Medical practice, I had repeatedly observed that overweight adults tended to be quite intelligent and able to process good information, when they could get it, resulting in correct conclusions. Most also tended to be aware of their weight problem and its implications. They seemed to be appropriately concerned about the weight accumulation and it's negative health effects, although often unwilling to admit this concern privately to anyone but a doctor. However, when provided with reliable information, overweight people can generally be depended on to make self benefiting and good decisions, even to the extent of changing their life styles and eating habits, sometimes alone, sometimes with Medical or other coaching help.

Some time ago, after multiple interviews with overweight men and women, it became apparent to me that something was almost uniquely wrong with those patients, most of whom were using the exact phrase "I don't eat that much" and I wondered why. Clearly, if one were to pay attention only to the body signal saying "I need food!" the individual could be expected to eat, and think he or she was behaving appropriately. However, if the signal from the stomach to the brain had been erroneous, or misinterpreted, the most readily understandable response would be simply to eat, with its inevitable consequence.

Further, if the mechanism for signaling had been faulty or misinterpreted, and the response had been eating, the long term result would be obesity, which explains the consequent attitude: "I don't eat that much (since I only eat when I'm hungry)". It is this concept that I advance in this small volume. It is my sincere hope that individuals who struggle with the results of overeating can gain enough understanding from this material and enough insight into their bodies' signals to be able to ignore the frequently erroneous signal saying "I need food!"

Nutrition is not a simple subject. But an understanding of the way the body handles its food supply and some of the things that can go wrong in that process is critical to developing insight into weight control. This is particularly true if one is relying only on internal sensations. Acquiring some knowledge of the body's method of handling the various types of foods we present to it daily may also provide some peace of mind to those who have succeeded at first, only later to fail to maintain a lower weight.

The thinking behind this book, and the purpose of adding yet another volume to the already crowded general library shelf on nutrition, particularly as it relates to being overweight, is to sort through and describe some of the established and well known facts in this troubling area. By doing so, I hope to promote a broader general understanding of the processes involved in digestion and nutrition. Coincidentally, I hope to be able to correct some of the more widely spread misunderstandings or outright fallacies that have developed or been put forward from time to time. However, many of the "facts" one hears all too often are not really facts, but unproven hypotheses, suppositions and conjectures, frequently inferred or built up from animal studies.

Probably the most important falsehood which occurs in this area is the one alluded to in this book's title. As we get into and try to understand some of the admittedly complex chemistry, anatomy, and physiology involved, we will begin to appreciate why our stomachs become unreliable in pointing out our bodies' desire (as opposed to need) for food. Unfortunately, a basic understanding of the chemical and physiologic principles involved is absolutely necessary to comprehend basic nutrition. Although I have tried to present this information without erroneous oversimplification, the complex interrelationships to be described sometimes defy simplification.

Over the years, many partially true propositions have been advanced with some justification. Usually, these propositions, although partially true, are incomplete and ignore another important part of nutritional physiology which invalidates the (false) conclusions being drawn. A few of these propositions will be treated herein, but since the limits of human invention (and greed) have never been defined, no attempt to deny fallacious claims already made or yet to be made can ever hope to be comprehensive, so I dare not even try. Although the basic organic chemistry and human physiology involved can be forbiddingly complex, I will try to simplify it enough to provide a basis for a better general layman's understanding of nutrition, while giving the reader enough information to allow the rejection of false claims.

Reviewing the contents provides an overview of the book's plan. Each chapter is designed to stand alone and to be understood for the most part without referring to the other chapters. This should be especially helpful for those readers who tend to break out in a rash, or worse, when confronted with chemical formulas. However, while not presuming to be a complete coverage of either nutritional physiology or of gastrointestinal anatomy or physiology, I hope to shed enough light on the underlying facts to provide the troubled reader with a basis on which to lay the resolve to cope with an overnourishment problem. Accordingly, some of the information, particularly about energy sources and energy utilization, will be essential to this understanding.

In the first part (Chapters 1—8), we present some of the chemical aspects of nutrition and energy. In the second part (Chapters 9—17), we describe some of the anatomy and physiology involved. Using the background thus provided, we will try to present in the third part (Chapters 18—21) some of the known, inferred or suspected features of nutrition. This well established information, with some of the physiologic unknowns, has led to much of the mystery and misery of weight misinformation. In the final part, I also attempt to respond to some of the more broadly made, outrageous or exasperating nutritional and pop-psychological misclaims, acknowledging at the outset that no attempt in this area can ever hope to be complete.

When the reader truly understands the substance of the book, he/she will understand also the corollary proposition to its title: "The scales usually don't lie", and be much better prepared to achieve and maintain a healthy weight and to evaluate false claims, frequently made out of context.

Good Luck!

Part One

Chemistry and Hidden Energy

Chapter 1

Organic Chemistry Concepts: Atoms and Molecules; Bonds and Energy Storage; 1, 2, and 3 Carbon Molecules; Longer Carbon Chains; Ketones, Carbonic Acid Termini and Carbonic Acids; Glycerol and Fatty Acids; Larger Acids; Rings; Basic Steroids; Isomerism

Atoms & Molecules

Almost as soon as we learn to read, we are given some understanding of chemistry, or "that branch of physical science which deals with several elementary substances of which all bodies are composed" (Oxford English Dictionary). Although the details are only considered later, the fact that everything in our expanding world is composed of tiny atoms or combinations of them is, at first, very hard to believe. Our developing sense of the physical world rebels. Still later, we become acquainted with the concept of atoms and are told that we are to be confronted with an entirely new alphabet set of one or two letters which will represent and correspond to those elemental atoms. Sodium (Na), Potassium (K), Chlorine (C), and Nitrogen (N) are a few members of our new Atomic Alphabet. Combinations, or gatherings, of the tiny atoms form larger, but still submicroscopic, molecules. Each of the molecules is composed of two or more of those atoms. We learn that the water we all become familiar with very early in life is a gathering of many atoms of two Hydrogen (H) and one Oxygen (O) atoms, combined into a number of single molecules (*Fig. 1.1a*). Much later, we are told that Chemistry has two main divisions. "Organic" Chemistry is the study of all molecules containing, at least, one Carbon (C) atom. "Inorganic" Chemistry is the study of all the other atoms and molecules. We also learn that the various molecular combinations of atoms can change or be made to change back and forth, but that the basic building blocks (nuclei) of those chemicals, the atoms, do not change. For the most part, the study of either of the main branches of chemistry is the study of these changes, the conditions under which they can be made to occur, the requirement of the presence of other substances or factors before a change can take place, and other variations. Diagrams are the easiest way to represent the atoms and molecules, and one or more lines drawn between the several letters representing the individual atoms are meant to show a connection between those particular atoms (*Figs. 1.1a and 1.1b*), called bonds. Here we have diagrams of those two common molecules.

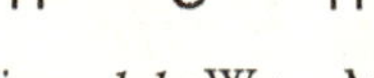

$$H\!-\!O\!-\!H \qquad\qquad\qquad O\!=\!C\!=\!O$$

Figure 1.1a Water Molecule   *Figure 1.1b* Carbon Dioxide Molecule
(Liquid at room temperature, H_2O)   (Gas, at room temperature, CO_2)

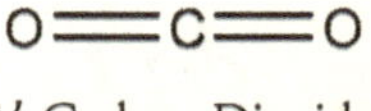

In order to better understand weight and weight control, an understanding of the basics of nutrition is essential. But before that, we need to try to understand the underlying chemical principles of nutrition. Therefore, we will start with the simplest carbon compounds. As is the Chemistry custom, this book uses the standard abbreviations, usually single capital letters, for the most common atoms, and simple lines to indicate the usual bonds between each atom within the various molecules.

Starting with a single Carbon atom, which usually has the ability to bond with four other single atoms we will use four lines extending from a Carbon atom to represent the usual connections between each Carbon atom ("C") and a same or different adjacent atom (*Fig. 1.2a*).

Bonds and Energy Storage

Since potential energy is stored within interatomic chemical bonds, we also first need to consider how the atoms are strung or bonded together. A bond existing between adjacent atoms, although a highly complex subject itself, is usually represented by a single line drawn between symbols for the two atoms. Stronger bonds exist, frequently representing greater energy storage or energy potential, and they are usually indicated by double lines between the atomic symbols. Very high energy storage intramolecular and interatomic bonds also exist and are usually indicated by the use of three lines between molecules. Later we learn that when one double bond occurs between two adjacent Carbon atoms in a longer carbon chain, the molecule is called "unsaturated". When more than one double bond is found between several carbon atoms in a much longer carbon chain, the molecule is said to be polyunsaturated. It was found possible to reduce the unsaturated doubled bonds between adjacent carbon atoms in unsaturated chains by a process called "saturation". "Hydrogenation" is the term used for this process by which liquid vegetable oils are converted to solid or cooking fats, similar to lard.

Structures:
One Carbon Molecules

Plain organic molecules can be as simple as a single carbon atom (*Fig. 1.2a*, the methyl compounds) with four hydrogen atoms bonded to it (*Fig. 1.2b*, methane gas). The insertion of an oxygen atom between a carbon atom and one of the hydrogen atoms creates an hydroxyl group or alcohol (*Fig. 1.3c*). Usually the hydroxyl group is bonded to a Carbon atom, but it may be attached to another atom. In the case of the single carbon molecule it forms methyl (or wood) alcohol (*Fig. 1.2c*), the permanent brain toxin. All these substances can be written out in diagrammatic form, using lines between the letters to represent the bonds between the atoms, as:

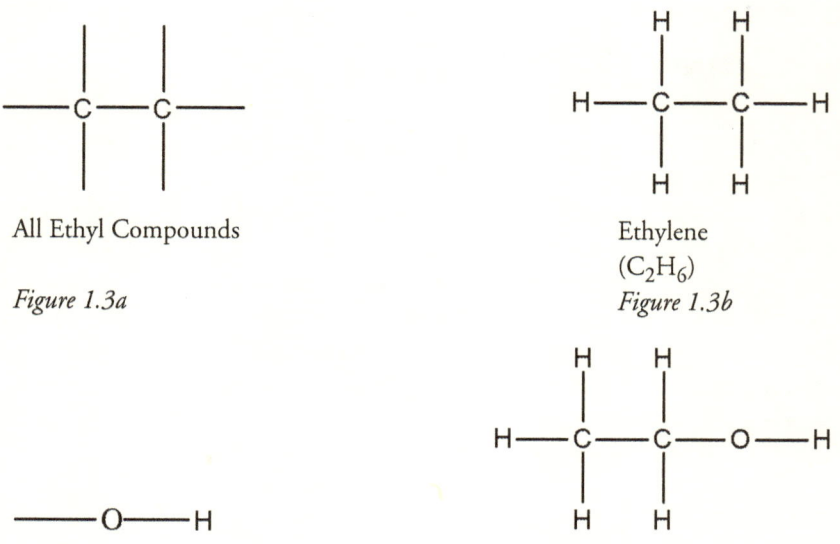

All Methyl Compounds
(only 1 Carbon)
Figure 1.2a

Methane:
(Gas, CH_4)
Figure 1.2b

Methyl Alcohol:
(Wood Alcohol, CH_3OH)
Figure 1.2c

Two and Three Carbon Chains

Two linked Carbon atoms or short chains exist and these molecules also can be completed only with hydrogen atoms (such compounds are called hydrocarbons; for examples see *Figs. 1.2b* and *1.3b*). Again, insertion of an oxygen atom between a carbon and hydrogen atom creates another hydroxyl group or alcohol (*Fig. 1.3c*) and in the case of two carbon atoms, ethyl alcohol (*Fig. 1.3d*). For comparison, although it is not nutritionally relevant, below is an example of another common, non-nutritional carbohydrate, Ethylene Glycol (antifreeze, *Fig. 1.3e*):

All Ethyl Compounds

Figure 1.3a

Ethylene
(C_2H_6)
Figure 1.3b

Figure 1.3c Hydroxyl Group
General Formula for "Alcohols"

Figure 1.3d Ethyl Alcohol (Common
Intoxicant, C_2H_6O) or (EtOH)

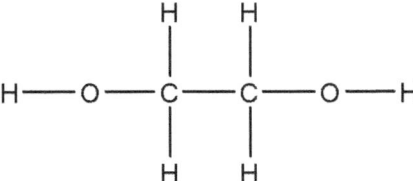

Figure 1.3e Ethylene Glycol (antifreeze)
$(C_2H_6O_2)$

Likewise, chains of three carbon molecules exist, but here, and hence upwards in numbers, the story becomes increasingly complex. A three carbon chain forms the basic structure of the "propyl" group of compounds (*Figs. 1.4a* and *1.4b*). If one oxygen atom is attached to the middle carbon atom, between it and one of it's hydrogen atoms, and an hydroxyl group (*Fig. 1.3c*) is thereby formed, the ends of the molecule are alike, and the molecule is called "isopropyl (or rubbing) alcohol" (*Fig. 1.4c*). If, on the other hand, an oxygen atom is inserted between a terminal carbon atom and one of its hydrogen atoms, again forming an hydroxyl group, the compound is called plain "propyl alcohol" (*Fig. 1.4d*). Thus:

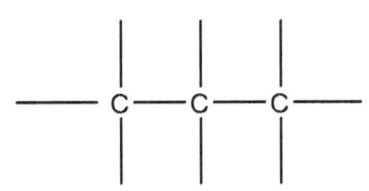

All Propyl Compounds
Figure 1.4a

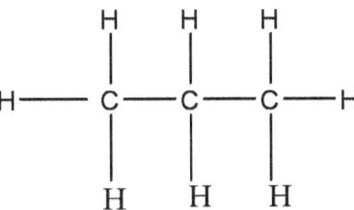

Propane
(C_3H_8)
Figure 1.4b

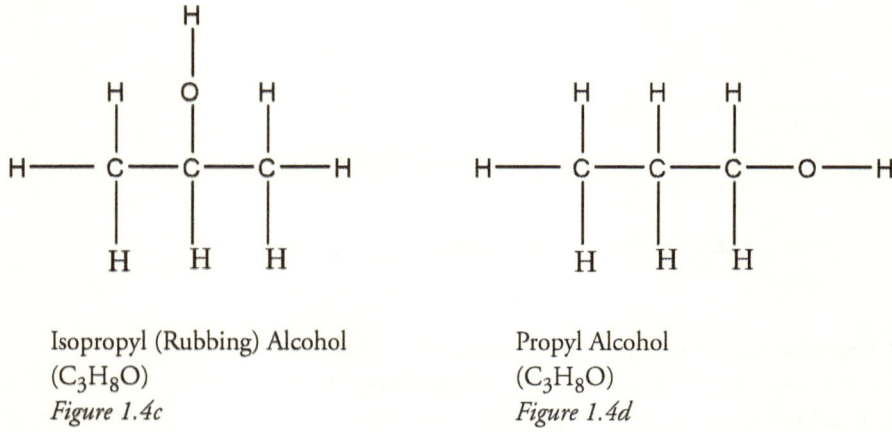

Isopropyl (Rubbing) Alcohol
(C_3H_8O)
Figure 1.4c

Propyl Alcohol
(C_3H_8O)
Figure 1.4d

Another, shorter system exists for writing organic formulae, called "empiric" but it is subject to misunderstanding. In the shorter system only the total numbers of each atom in a molecule is given, thus methane is CH_4, methyl alcohol is CH_4O, ethane is C_2H_6, ethyl alcohol C_2H_6O, etc. For the first few molecules we also provide empiric formulae. However, both propyl and isopropyl alcohol are C_3H_8O. Although the system is very convenient and widely used, because of overlaps like those occurring between propyl and isopropyl alcohol, it can be confusing. Another common shorthand occurs when the naming systems are combined, for instance "acute ET(hyl)OH(alcohol) TOX(icity)" is Medical shorthand for drunk!

Longer Carbon Chains

We now will skip up the carbon atom chain to consider six linear linked carbon atoms, the basic sugars (See Chapter 2). Although there are shorter and longer chained sugars, they are not very significant nutritionally. Typically, Fatty Acids consist of longer Carbon chains, some of which have unsaturated intercarbon bonds (*Fig. 4.3*). Most of the sugars have a single bond and depend on the angle of attachment between the carbon, oxygen, and hydrogen atoms for their unique molecular structure, function, properties, and names. For instance, glucose and galactose each contain the same number of atoms ($C_6H_{14}O_6$), but physiologically behave very differently. Shorter chained sugars exist, but since the body can make them all they are not nutritionally as important, although they undoubtedly participate in the body's chemistry.

Since most physiologic chemical reactions occur around carbon atoms, the hydrogen atoms are usually ignored in representations, but it is generally understood that, in reality, they are there. In addition, the particular carbon atoms that are usually the site of activity in any physiologic chemical reaction are frequently targeted by the presence of another group on one carbon in a structure (see below). Less frequently, another type of atom, sulfur (S), phosphorous (P), nitrogen (N) (see Proteins in Chapter 3), or other may be an attachment point for a different molecule or chain. Sometimes many (even thousands) mostly 6-carbon sugars will be found linked. These comprise the dietary starches (of both animal and vegetable origin) that must be broken down into their components before their stored, potential energy can be digested, absorbed, and then used.

Ketones

We also must consider the case of an oxygen atom doubly bonded to a carbon atom, called a ketone (*Fig.1.5*):

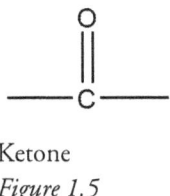

Ketone
Figure 1.5

In the body's wonderful chemical factory, ketones (or so the class of ketone bearing chains is called) are frequently converted back and forth to various types of hydroxyl groups (alcohols) or acids, but the oxygen usually remains attached to its carbon.

Carbonic Acids and Carbonic Acid Termini

Another important part of the body's chemistry is the presence of a ketone and an hydroxyl group together on a single carbon atom (*Fig. 1.6*). This is usually represented in this way:

Carbonic Acid Terminus

Figure 1.6

When a ketone occurs on a single carbon with an attached hydroxyl (the words atom or group are frequently dropped, but understood) the compound is called Carbonic Acid (Fig. 1.7a). Although the double ketone bond is a part of the acidic terminus, the acid effect is more prominent, hence any chain with this ending is called an acid. Longer Carbon chains bearing this configuration at one end are all called "acids". Using another chemical convention, the "R" in this diagram (Fig. 1.7b) refers to a longer chain of Carbon atoms (see Chapter 4 on Fatty Acids).

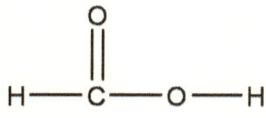

Carbonic Acid (H2CO2)

Figure 1.7a

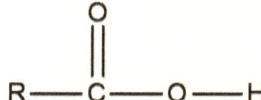

Generic Formula for Organic Acids

Figure 1.7b (R=any carbon chain, 1 or more)

Glycerol and Fatty Acids

Before considering other higher number carbon compounds, we need to be aware of another nutritionally important 3 carbon and 3 hydroxyl compound, called glycerol (*Figs. 1.8 & 1.9a*). At their oxygen atoms, each of the 3 carbon atoms of glycerol provide anchors, or points of attachment, for particular longer chained substances called "fatty acids" (*Fig. 1.9b*). This combination, when it exists, makes a complete fat molecule, also-called a "triglyceride" (*Fig. 1.9c*). The body, in its wonderful capacity as a chemical factory, can make glycerol and most of the fatty acids, and, once the fatty acids are made, complete fats can be formed by attaching 3 fatty acids to the glycerol (See Chapter 4), and releasing three molecules of water in the process (*Fig. 1.9d*).

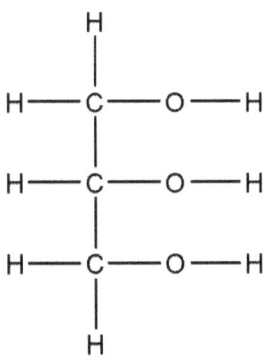

Glycerol ($C_3H_8O_3$)
Figure 1.8

Since organic acids usually attach to glycerol's carbon atoms via an oxygen linking atom, the most common representation of glycerol is as a triple hydroxyl alcohol, as presented in more detail in Chapter 4, thus:

The components of a fat molecule are:

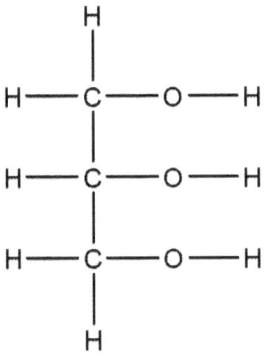

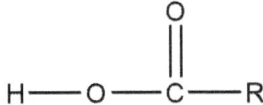

Glycerol Portion
of Fat Molecule
Figure 1.9a

3 different Fatty Acids Portion
of Fat Molecule
R (any Carbon chain), may be R_1, R_2 and R_3
Figure 1.9b

And, when combined, look like *Fig. 1.9c*:

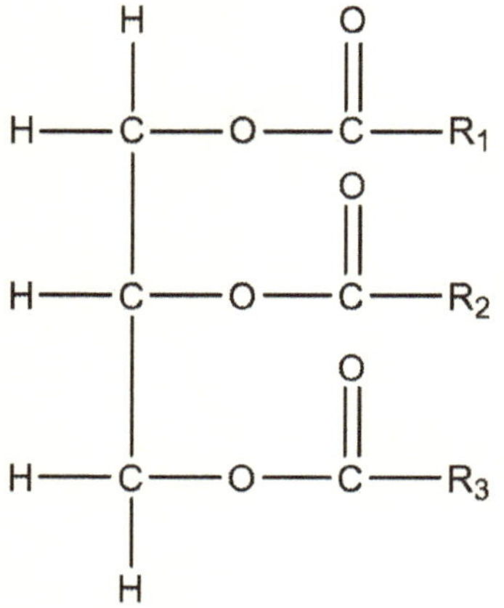

Generic Formula for Fat (see Chapter IV Fats)
Figure 1.9c (and *Figure 4.2*)

$+3$ H——O——H

Extra Water Molecules Produced by
Formation of a single Fat Molecule
Figure 1.9d

Although they can be different from each other on a complete fat molecule, the Fatty Acids attached to one Glycerol can be all of the same type (i.e.$R_1=R_2=R_3$). Each combination of a Fatty Acid with one of the hydroxyl branches of a Glycerol molecule produces one molecule of Water (*Fig. 1.9d*).

Jumping way ahead in our story of nutritional chemistry, here we briefly consider complete fats, which are more fully considered in Chapter 4. Fatty acids are usually composed of longer carbon chains, and are usually represented generically as "R," e.g. R1, R2, R3, etc. for different fatty acids (*Fig. 1.9b* and *1.9c*), although they could probably be labeled more accurately as "FA1, FA2, FA3". Thus, diagrammatically, when a complete fat molecule is formed, the formula might look like that presented in *Figure 4.2*, or here, as in *Figure 1.9c*.

Larger Acids

Again, a longer chain of carbon atoms, combined with other atoms, can occur by combining with glycerol or by attaching to the carbon on another carbonic acid terminus, or elsewhere. Not as strong as some of the more robust acids, like hydrochloric (HCl) or sulfuric (H_2SO_4), the carbonic fatty acid terminus is nevertheless acidic and usually reacts with bases by donating a hydrogen atom to the hydroxyl (or-OH part) of the base to form a separate molecule of water (H_2O), and, in the process, it becomes bonded to the base remaining.

The carbonic acid part of a larger or more complex molecule may also be the point of attachment of another molecular fragment. Much larger molecules (proteins, for instance) may bear an acidic complex at one location in their structure, while bearing a base (the opposite of an acid) in another area. These two active parts of one molecule may react to each other and interconnect (forming a ring) if the adjacent carbon chain is sufficiently long and flexible enough to allow them to touch.

The connections between atoms in many organic molecules are, for the most part, stable, although after consumption and digestion, with conversion by the body for food energy, other new, smaller molecules undoubtedly are formed. Potential energy is usually liberated from the breaking down of molecules, most of which have been consumed from external sources. It is in the complex chemical processes attendant upon and preceding consumption of these external energy sources that our bodies tend to mislead us (see Chapter 18). Nevertheless the energy requirements and production for each chemical reaction, although individually quite miniscule, are also firmly fixed, inviolate and, therefore, mandatory, as are the energy and variety supplied in this manner from various food sources.

As a more efficient way of storing energy, bonds between atoms are made weaker, but with higher potential energy storage by doubling or even tripling the linkage. Indeed, one of the most commonly used reactions for energy storage and release is provided by movement between a particular double and triple bond structure.

Whenever the available energy taken in by an organism exceeds that currently needed for upkeep (or basic metabolism), a method for temporary energy storage may be used by the body. By constructing an entire molecule based on the three carbon glycerol combining with multiple unsaturated fatty acids, more efficient energy storage with space conservation is achieved. Since humans are basically another form of animal (speaking physiologically or chemically), and since animals tend to store energy in single bonded (or "saturated") forms of the fatty acids, human and animal fats tend to be of the saturated variety. Plants, on the other hand, and some fish tend to store energy in multi-bonded (or "unsaturated") fatty acids (See Chapter 4).

Ring Structures:
Carbon

Before leaving the subject of bonds, it is also important to consider a few of the ring structures. The mystery of figuring out how six carbon atoms could possibly be accompanied by only six hydrogen atoms in benzene (C_6H_6) was worked out in the mid-1800's by determining that the carbon atoms were linked together in a ring. The so-called benzene ring, is usually represented thus, with three double and three single bonds between the carbon atoms (*Figs .1.10a & 1.10b*):

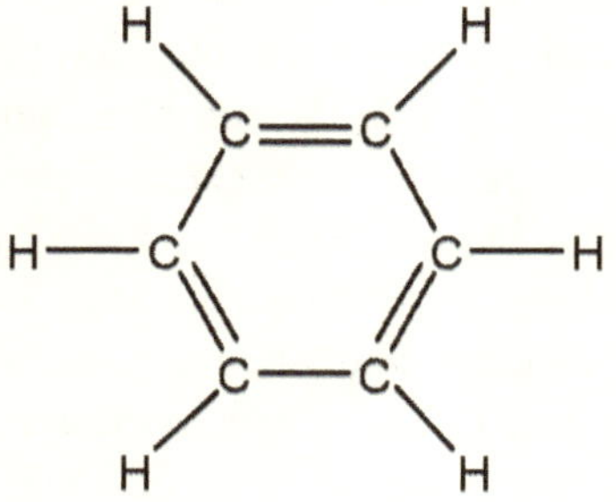

Benzene (C_6H_6)
Figure 1.10a

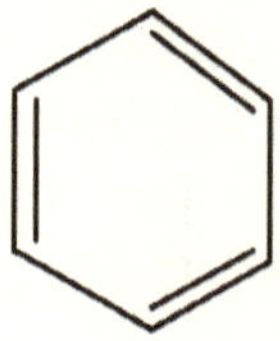

Benzene (as usually drawn)
Figure 1.10b

When an hydroxyl group is added to the benzene molecule it becomes a molecule of phenol, or Benzene alcohol (*Fig. 1.11*). In concentrated form, this substance is caustic, but diluted, it also participates in the formation of many non-caustic organic molecules, some of major nutritional interest.

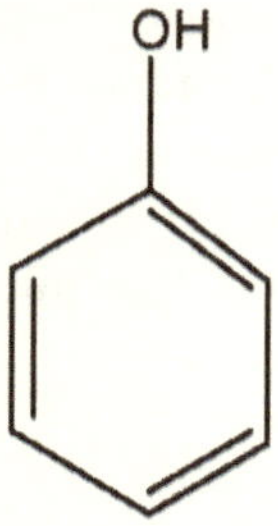

Phenol (C_6H_6O)
Figure 1.11

Nitrogen

Similarly, nitrogen participates in some ring structures, although this ring usually contains only five atoms, one of which is the nitrogen, the other four being carbon (*Figs. 1.12a* and *1.12b*). Since another type of atom is involved, it is not truly a carbohydrate, but if nitrogen is the added component, any substance bearing this ring qualifies as an amino acid, peptide, or protein.

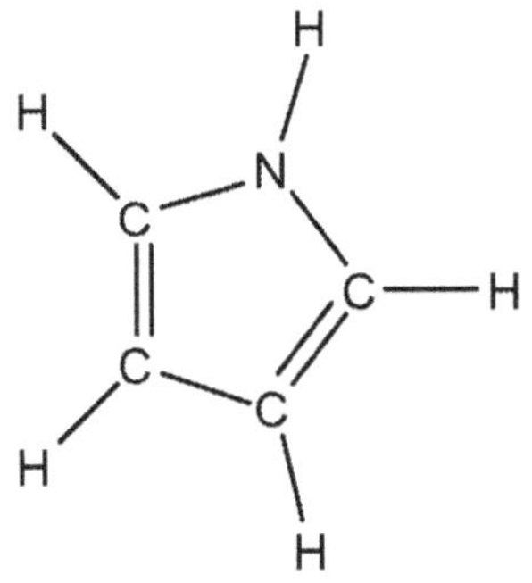

Pyrrole Ring
Figure 1.12a

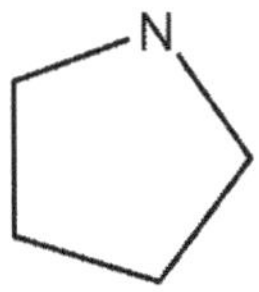

Pyrrole Ring (as usually drawn)
Figure 1.12b

Many other ring structures occur, some involving other atoms than nitrogen.

The Basic Steroid Ring

Another ring structure that is physiologically very significant is the basic so-called steroid ring. Since many of the hormones (See Chapter 15), cholesterol (which the body is able to manufacture), and other chemicals are based on various attachments to this 17-carbon structure and its several specific side chains, its importance cannot be overemphasized. The basic Steroid molecule contains four saturated rings with one or two hydrogen atoms bound to each carbon atom (Rings labeled here):

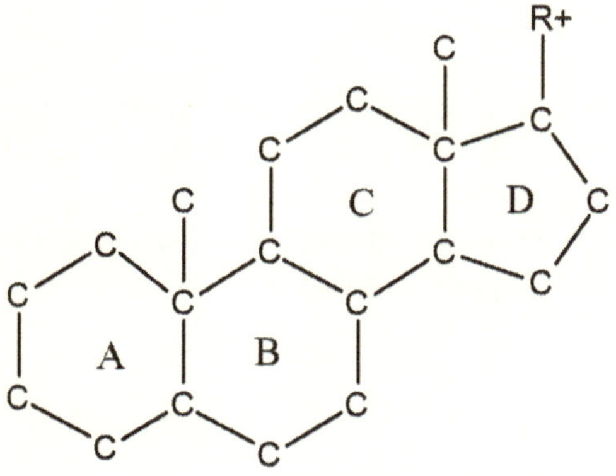

Figure 1.13
(For Standard Carbon Numbering See *Figure 4.5*, Hydrogen atoms understood)

In the steroid ring the individual carbon atoms are identified by numbering (as seen in *Fig. 4.5*), and variations in the ring structure and some of the most important places of attachments are indicated in Chapter 4. Frequently omitted entirely from the structural diagrams (as here), are the hydrogen atoms. Unless otherwise noted, all bonds in the steroid nucleus are saturated.

The longer chain structures, as well as the rings, apparently fold over and even back upon themselves, although in diagrammatic representation they are presented as flat. Actually they are more like folded chains which can go in many directions, but must follow certain inviolate rules, particularly in chemical reactions. Pure starch compounds are usually made up of strings of many (thousands) of 6-carbon molecules.

Isomerism

Sometimes it helps, in trying to visualize chemical structures of similar composition, to picture oneself in the position of one of the carbon atoms. When we do this from the standpoint of any particular atom in a simple sugar linear chain we can see that some of the adjacent carbons will be pointing off in one direction while others with the very same contents, and looking at them from the very same vantage point, will be pointing off in an entirely different direction. If the carbon chains are dissimilar (not the case with the propyl compounds, but true of the higher number carbon molecules), there will be more than one possible configuration or physical structure of the molecule. When solutions of molecules with similar components and almost the same structure are separated, they can cause polarized light passed through a solution of them to rotate. An even mixture of right-handed and left-handed light rotating structures is said to be "racemic", and, in solution, will not cause polarized light to rotate. However, the rotating ability is found whenever a molecule contains a carbon atom with four different atomic attachments, e.g.-H,-OH,-O, or a carbon chain (upwards from two). This simple fact apparently accounts for the wide variation in the metabolic characteristics of otherwise quite similar structures. Interestingly, most naturally occurring substances are levorotary, their solutions rotating polarized light to the left. Why? No adequate explanation exists, but it might have to do with the earth's rotation.

Chapter 2

Carbohydrates: Simple and Complex Sugars, Complex Intolerance, Starches and "Fiber," Carbohydrate Energy, Alcohol, Intercarbohydrate Conversion, Plant-Animal Complimentarity

Carbohydrates

In order to achieve a basic understanding of nutrition, we must first consider the class of food chemicals called "Carbohydrates". This class of organic compounds is defined by all the molecules being composed exclusively of carbon, hydrogen, and oxygen atoms. We differentiate between "Hydrocarbons" and carbohydrates since the former contain only hydrogen and carbon atoms. Consequently, the common gas Carbon Dioxide (*Fig. 1.1b*, AKA dry ice), is not, strictly speaking, either one. All the simpler forms of carbohydrates are manufactured within the body and are made by the body's wonderful chemical machinery only from those three atomic elements, carbon (C), hydrogen (H), and oxygen (O), as we saw in Chapter 1. Although at first glance, these reactions appear quite simple, the body seems to be able to manufacture whatever larger carbohydrate molecules it needs from the foods presented to it. At least to date, none of the carbohydrates have been found "essential" (as defined in Chapter 8).

Simple Sugars

In addition to the simple compounds mentioned above, the simple sugars (amyloses) are composed of short chains of carbon atoms (usually 3 to 8). Usually the sugar carbons contain a bond to an adjacent hydrogen atom on one side, and each usually contains an hydroxyl group (*Fig. 1.3c*) on the side opposite to the single hydrogen in a long carbon chain. The empiric formulae for the simple sugars are thus: $C_3H_8O_3$, trioses; $C_4H_{10}O_4$, tetroses; $C_5H_{12}O_5$, pentoses; and $C_6H_{14}O_6$, hexoses etc. (*Figs. 2.1a. 2.1b, 2.1c*):

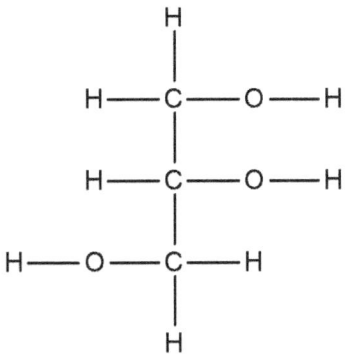

An Example of a Triose ($C_3H_8O_3$)
Figure 2.1a

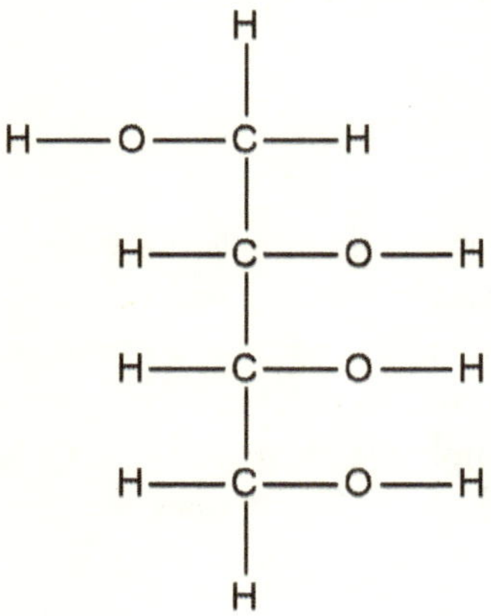

An example of a Tetrose ($C_4H_{10}O_4$)
Figure 2.1b

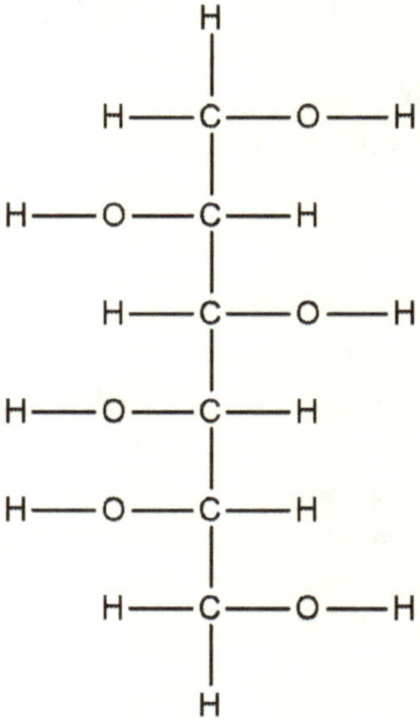

An example of an Hexose ($C_6H_{14}O_6$)
Figure 2.1c

Larger Molecules, including Complex Sugars

Longer chained and more complex molecules are manufactured both in animals and plants from the shorter chains by chemically linking some of the simple sugars together. This process may even start by the linking together of some two carbon structures, which are produced when ingested food substances are broken down or digested within the intestine and then absorbed into the blood stream. The simpler sugar molecules are usually presented to each animal (herbivore or not) in one of these larger forms. By the various linking of two simple six carbon sugars together, a different twelve carbon, or complex sugar structure is created. Depending on the linkage, the particular combination, and composition, as well as the source, sucrose, lactose, maltose, or some other of the more complex sugars may be formed (*Fig. 2.2*). Thus, a combination of galactose and glucose forms lactose, or milk sugar, with unique intercarbon connections, etc.

Cellulose: Glucose and Glucose (Fiber, indigestible in humans)
Maltose: Glucose and Glucose (Humanly digestible)
Lactose: Glucose and Galactose (Milk Sugar)
Sucrose: Glucose and Fructose (Table Sugar)

Some examples of 12 Carbon sugars (combinations of 6 Carbon sugars)
Figure 2.2

The digestive process requires the breaking down or reversal of those processes by which the various food molecules are formed, before the contained energy can be absorbed.

Unavailability and Intolerance to Complex Sugars

Apart from Cellulose, when the digestive process is deficient in the intestinal secretion of the specific enzyme needed to separate the higher sugars into their components before they can be absorbed, intolerance to that particular sugar is said to exist in the individual so afflicted (e.g. the common Mediterranean and African trait of lactose intolerance). In the Lactose Intolerance Syndrome undigested lactose within the intestinal lumen draws water into the Gut to dilute the unabsorbed lactose, thus causing the crampy diarrhea of that syndrome. Since the normal human digestive system is unable to break down some of the bonds that form the various celluloses, the smaller molecules of which they are made are unavailable to the human energy cycle. Although some animals can break down and then absorb the sugars in cellulose, all humanly indigestible cellulose is simply called "fiber".

Starches and "Fiber"

By forming combinations of sugars in various manners, a much greater number of structures containing only Carbon, Hydrogen, and Oxygen (literally thousands of types of molecules) are formed. Similarly, other complex structures are formed with the primary component being one of the basic carbohydrates or starches, however another element, or atom, frequently participates in those formations. Therefore, at least when a different atom is involved, they become, no longer, strictly speaking, carbohydrates.

Digestible starch is formed by various members of the plant kingdom and is composed of long linear chains of simple sugars (amyloses) and branched chains of simple sugars (amylopectins). Animals manufacture and store their sugars in a branched chain molecule called "glycogen" or animal starch. Similarly, the humanly indigestible (but widespread in the plant kingdom) cellulose, or fiber, is composed primarily of sugar based structures. Cellulose is humanly indigestible because of cross linkages between several of the simple sugars within its molecular structure. (Cows and other herbivores that subsist solely on plants can normally digest and use these substances without difficulty.) Even though we humans can neither digest nor derive any energy from it, cellulose, or "fiber", is an important part of our diet because it adds "bulk". In as much as humans do not derive any energy from cellulose, like water, it is calorically neutral. The concept of Caloric neutrality excepts the energy utilized in the eating and the smooth muscle exertion spent in propelling the cellulose downwards within the intestine. However, plant fiber, or cellulose, is thought to have some additional beneficial effects, particularly in cancer avoidance. Cellulose constitutes a very significant part of the molecular plant kingdom structure (e.g. vegetables and fruits) and is a large part of many of the foods we normally consume. Other forms of carbohydrates exist in nature, although they are of less nutritional concern.

Much has been made of the difference between "simple" sugars and "complex" carbohydrates or "carbs". Actually, when digested and absorbed (excluding cellulose) these substances have exactly the same amount of caloric or nutritional value on a per dry gram basis, differing only slightly in the speed with which the digestive enzymes prepare them for absorption within the intestinal lumen (see Chapters 9-17 on digestion).

Carbohydrate Energy (Calories)

In deriving energy from that stored within the various usable starch chemicals, one finds that approximately four Kilocalories (Calories for short) are produced from each gram of starch used or stored by the body for energy. (A physical unit called "Calorie" is the amount of thermal energy or heat required to raise the temperature of a milliliter of water one degree, Centigrade, at sea level. A Kilocalorie is a thousand of them.) We use the word "Calorie" in place of "Kilocalorie" as a matter of custom and convenience, although the dietary usage of the word "Calorie" means a thousand actual thermal calories). So if we derive energy from a gram of simple 6-Carbon glucose or table sugar (sucrose) instead of a complex starch, we also gain four kilocalories (Calories in the conventional dietary meaning; see Kilocalories in Chapter 6). Thus, and these numbers are completely reliable, all starches and table sugar (or, strictly speaking, the "carbs" and simple sugars) have exactly the same caloric or potential energy value (the former only requiring another digestive or chemical breakdown step before absorption). Later, we will appreciate how this fact can be unintentionally or intentionally misused. Since the body's wonderful chemical factory can convert energy back and forth between the starches and sugars, none of the sugars are said to be "essential". However, while life exists with its ongoing need for caloric energy, there is a continuing requirement for the caloric or energy support these substances provide.

Ethyl Alcohol Energy

Another source of "carbohydrate" energy is that supplied by ethyl alcohol, although some prefer to consider this substance separately. In this exceptional case, seven Calories are derived per gram (there are approximately 15 grams of ethyl alcohol in a 30 ml. shot of 100 proof whisky and 4 grams of ethyl alcohol in 100 ml. of 4% beer, exclusive of the other Calorie yielding substances in this beverage). Since pure alcohol contains no other types of atoms, it is a carbohydrate by definition. Ingestion of ethyl alcohol allows the operation of both the temporary brain toxin and blood vessel dilation effects without losing any of its potential as a source of Calories or chemical energy as the two carbon structure is incorporated into the body's metabolism. (It is speculated that skin vasodilatation caused by alcohol and resultant body cooling is the source of the "so-called" warming sensation of whiskey. The actual effect is more rapid heat radiation from the body because of more body heat loss due to skin vessel dilatation, erroneously sensed as warmth).

Intercarbohydrate Conversion

The conversion back and forth between and among the various carbohydrates obviously becomes a highly complex biochemical subject. But the important thing for anyone struggling with attempted weight loss to understand is that this interconversion can and does occur without any conscious effort on anyone's part. The other very important concept, one of energy economy, relates to the body's tendency to retain currently unneeded ingested food energy for later use. Through mechanisms for supposedly temporary storage of ingested chemical energy, for later or emergency use, the body converts carbohydrate energy and creates and stores this energy in the most space efficient chemical way available to it, namely, in fats (see Chapter 4). Formerly, this process may well have had survival advantages in more harsh times. In modern times, with food readily available and our well fed life styles, the same tendency has now become a curse.

Plant-Animal Complimentarity

The complimentary metabolisms of the plant and animal kingdoms are nicely demonstrated by a consideration of the carbohydrates. When presented with water (H_2O) and carbon dioxide (CO_2), plants under the effect of sunlight, are able to manufacture the sugars, starches, and other energy supplies that we and the other members of the animal kingdom use. In the process of utilizing the carbohydrates, animals produce water and carbon dioxide, which in turn can be recycled again by plants as long as the sun continues to shine.

Chapter 3

Nitrogen containing Molecules: Amino Acids, Nomenclature, Enzymes, Peptides and Proteins, Digestion and Manufacture, Nitrogen Balance, Protein Energy and Sparing

Amino Acids

There are several (20 naturally occurring) small carbon molecules found in animals, each of which contains at least one Nitrogen atom. Because they each have a carbonic acid terminus at one extremity they are truly called acids, although they are very weak (*Fig. 3.1*). These tiny nitrogen containing molecules are called amino acids. They are the basic building blocks of a different class of food compounds, called peptides and proteins.

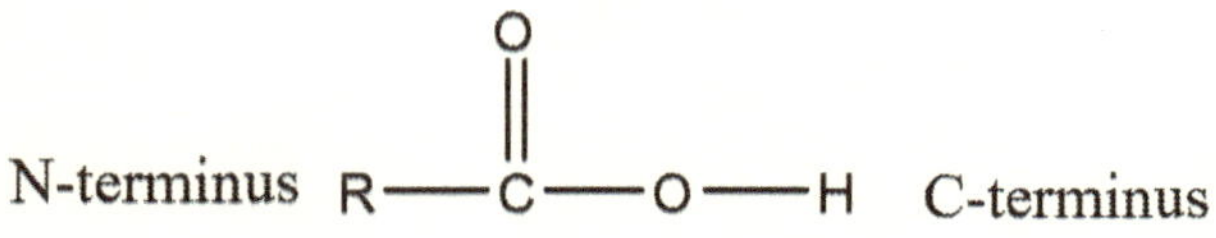

$$O$$
$$\|$$
N-terminus   R——C——O——H   C-terminus

Typical Amino Acid Naming System (Here the "R", or carbon chain, contains at least one Nitrogen Atom)
Figure 3.1

Smaller combinations of molecules made up of these amino acid molecules are called peptides while the larger combinations, called proteins, are made from many thousands of amino acids. Proteins may also contain other structures, some with great variation.

Because each amino acid bears at least one nitrogen atom, compounds made from them are excluded from the food class "carbohydrates". Amino Acids are a significant part of every animal diet and a part of all living structures, both plant and animal. In addition to the nitrogen, two of the amino acids also contain a sulfur atom and a few others contain phenolic rings. Because the human body cannot manufacture eleven of the amino acids they are called the "essential amino acids" (*Fig. 3.2* and Chapter 8). Since the body can manufacture almost all of the other compounds it needs to maintain its ongoing metabolism and life processes, many of the non-essential molecular structures are produced without any conscious direction on our part, as long as the basic molecular building blocks are on hand (i.e. supplied by the dietary intake) and available (*Fig. 3.3*). (This excludes and does not apply to "vitamins," which are considered in more depth in Chapter 7.)

Termini and Names

Because the acidic carbon atom is at one extremity of each amino acid molecule, peptide or protein, that end is referred to as the carbon or "C" terminus. The opposite or non-acidic (or non-C) end of each molecule is called the "N" terminus, although the nitrogen atom may not be exactly at the end of the molecular chain (*Fig. 3.1*). When several amino acids are linked into a larger peptide or protein structure C to N linkage can occur within the larger molecule, but the same (C & N) terminology applies.

Therefore, both peptides and the even larger protein molecules have both "C" and "N" termini. Proteins, frequently huge, are larger molecules made up from the nitrogen containing amino acids, either alone or in combination with other elements or structures. Proteins may be composed of one or more chains. Some proteins are entirely humanly indigestible (comparable to cellulose). These need not concern us when discussing potential energy or food values. Some special proteins are called "globulins," each with a unique function. Some members of the globulins are the various hemoglobins, responsible for carrying oxygen throughout the body, and the myoglobins that have unique contractile abilities.

Essential Amino Acids

Several of the amino acids cannot be manufactured by the body and must be included in the diet. For that reason they are called, and must be considered, "essential".

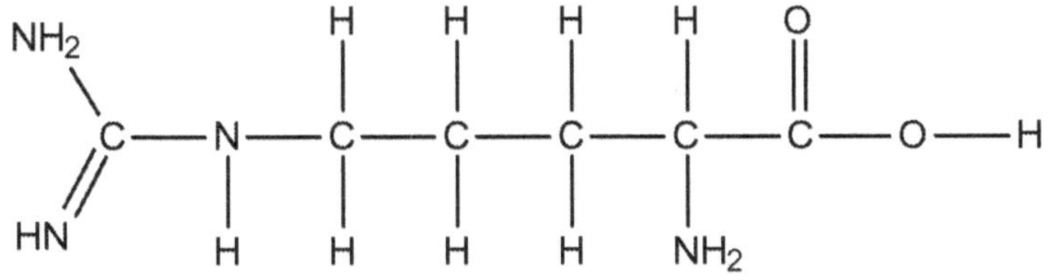

Arginine

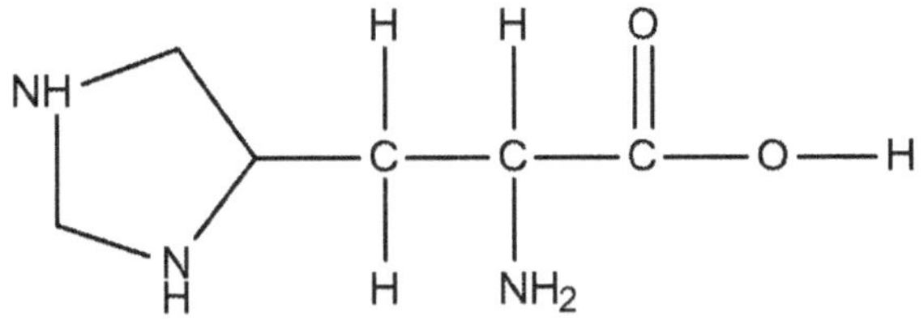

Histadine

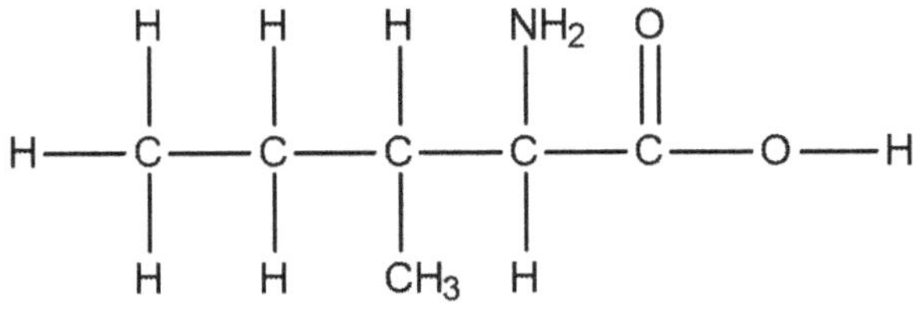

Isolucine

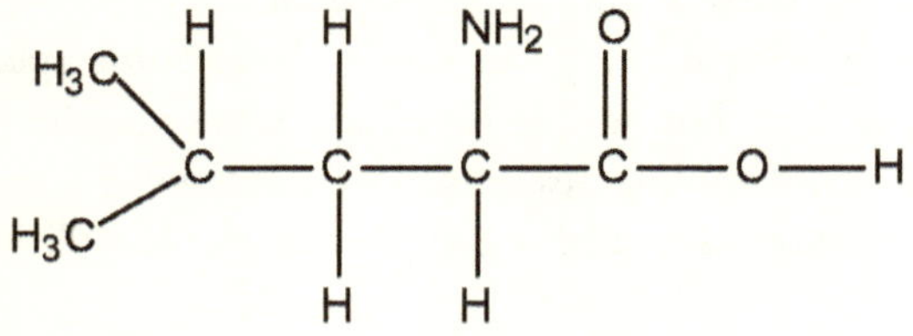

Leucine

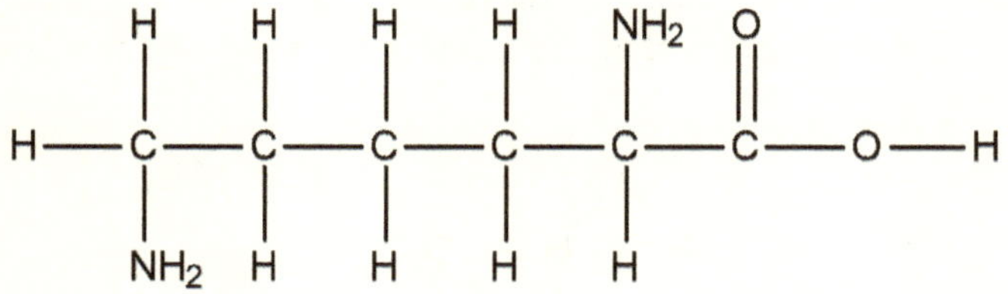

Lysine

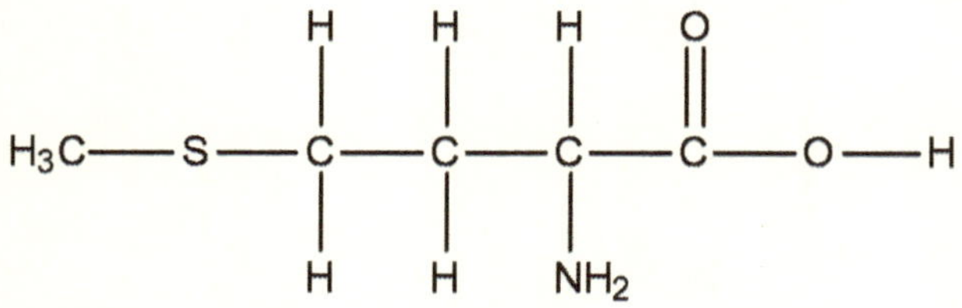

Methionine

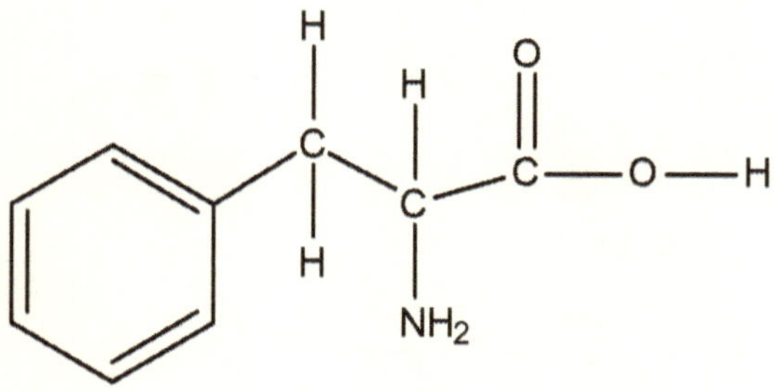

Phenylalanine

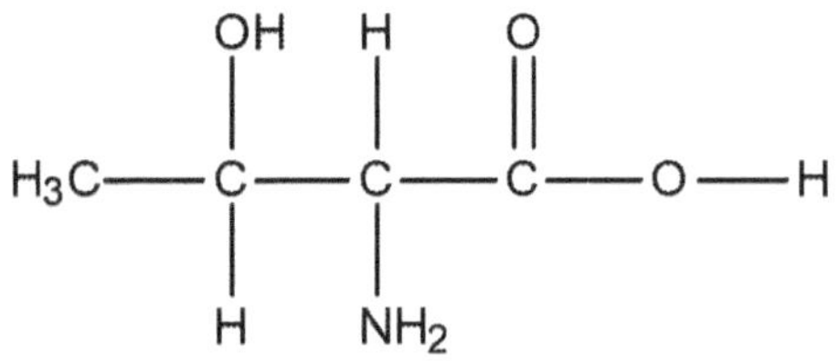

Threonine

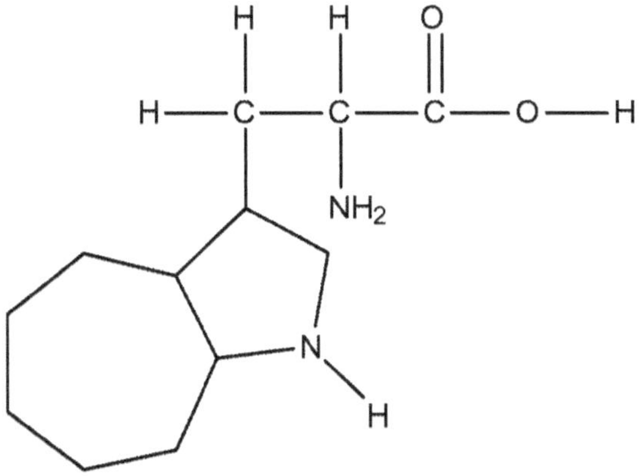

Tryptophane

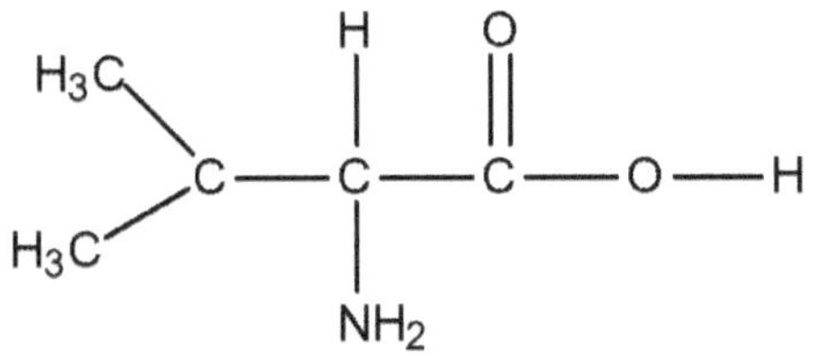

Valine

Figure 3.2 Essential Amino Acids List & Structures

Alanine ($C_3H_7O_2N$), Aspargine ($C_4H_8O_3N_2$), Aspartic Acid ($C_4H_7O_4N$), Cysteine ($C_3H_7O_2NS$), Dibromotyrosine ($C_9H_9O_3Br_2N$), Diiodotyrosine ($C_9H_9O_3I_2N$), Glutamic Acid ($C_4H_9O_4N$), Glutamine ($C_5H_{10}O_3N_2$), Glycine ($C_2H_5O_2N$), Hydroxylysine ($C_6H_{14}O_3N_2$), Hydroxyproline ($C_5H_5O_3N$), Proline ($C_5H_9O_2N$), Serine ($C_3H_7O_3N$), Thyroxine ($C_{15}H_{10}O_4I_4N$), Tyrosine ($C_9H_{11}O_3N$).

Figure 3.3 Names (and content) of Other (Non-essential) Natural Amino Acids

Although "Non-essential" amino acids are components of many proteins since they can be manufactured by the body, they are called not "essential" to be in the diet.

Peptides & Proteins

In a similar fashion to the mechanism by which the higher sugars and starches are built up from the simpler sugar molecules, peptides (with 2 to 100 or more various amino acid components) and proteins (with many more amino acids, and perhaps other components also), are formed by the linking up of two or more amino acids or one amino acid and another structure or structures (sugars or fatty acids). Some of the peptide molecules thus formed play a very active role in all animal metabolism; some participate in structure formation; some act simply as catalysts by participating in a reaction (or reactions) without being consumed in the reaction or ending up as a part of the final molecule. Amino acids participate in the formation of even larger molecules, called proteins. By convention, polypeptides have a molecular weight up to 10,000, proteins above that. Much of the finer points of amino acid and protein chemistry need not concern us here. It is sufficient to understand that the nitrogen part of each molecule endows these acids with unique and very physiologically useful features, justifying in part, their separate designation.

Complex Compounds

Indigestible fibers apparently do confer some health benefits, although most of the indigestible plant fibers are not proteins, but celluloses of various kinds (see

Chapter 2, Carbohydrates). On the other hand, as part of our study of nutrition we do need to know about some of the various special combinations of amino acid based structures with other, usually highly complex, molecules. Although, as with the other chemical structures, we represent these molecules in a linear or flat fashion for ease of consideration, we do so with the understanding that the longer molecules actually fold about and even double back on themselves and interconnect one or several times. Among the important proteins or protein combinations are skin and bone collagens, hemoglobin, myoglobin, and bile pigments, lipoproteins, and some enzymes. Although the several collagens are, for the most part, indigestible by humans, their formation and upkeep are vital to body function. The various hemoglobin molecules are an integral part of each body's ability to store, transport, and utilize oxygen within each cellular unit. The bile pigments are formed from the hemoglobin and myoglobin molecules and excreted after the body has extracted most of their contained iron atoms. The lipoproteins are combinations of proteins and various fat substances and are considered in the next chapter (4) on Lipids.

Enzymes

Enzymes are frequently found within the protein group and serve as facilitators of the many chemical reactions that are taking place continually within any living body. Although the enzymes must be present to facilitate these reactions, and although their participation is as vital to ongoing life as are their products, they are not consumed in the process nor included in the product, emerging from the reaction unchanged. Although many of the enzymes are proteins, others are not. Some vitamins are enzymes and cannot be manufactured by the body, thereby fulfilling the definitional requirement of "vitamin," or essential to ongoing life.

Protein Digestion and Manufacture

The processes by which the various compounds are broken down within the body are referred to collectively as "catabolism". However, when this happens within the intestinal lumen it is considered a part of the normal digestive process. Naturally, one of the end products of protein catabolism is nitrogen, and the methods by which the body handles the waste nitrogen of catabolism is another subject entirely. For our purposes, we will assume that the waste handling mechanisms are intact, although this is not a universally valid assumption. Another product of protein catabolism is the sulfur atom, which, when combined with hydrogen, forms the olfactorally offensive gas, hydrogen sulfide (H_2S). It is the H_2S odor that we associate with rotting tissue and flatus. The processes of protein breakdown are carried out within the gut lumen (but actually outside the body's internal environment) by the digestive catabolism of food chemicals within the gut. Absorption of the individual amino acids takes place into the internal environment after they are released. In reverse order to the processes by which peptides, then proteins, have been formed previously, during intestinal breakdown, the individual amino acids are cleaved from the larger molecules by the actions of the secretions of the digestive glands and the gut lining cells, or "mucosa," prior to their absorption. Once in the simpler form, these chemicals are absorbed by the gut lining cells and passed into the blood or lymph. After absorption the absorbed products provide either atomic or molecularly needed structures or potential chemical energy by being carried by the blood to wherever they are to be used, dissolved, or suspended in the blood serum. "Anabolism" is the name given to the general processes by which the body builds up and renews its various structures (e.g. growth, muscles, and organs) from the chemical components supplied in the diet after they have been broken down within the intestine and absorbed from the intestine or "digested" (the entire process). The amino acids or other compounds are then taken into each needy cell and incorporated into the body's structure or function.

Nitrogen Balance

If the dietary intake of protein is adequate, both in amount and variety of essential amino acids, and if nitrogen excretion approximates intake so that the needs of the body are being met daily or weekly, one is said to be in "Nitrogen Balance". This concept derives its importance from the fact that the body has little ability to store nitrogen for later use; not the case with pure chemical energy, or calories. If various foods do not contain all the essential amino acids, they are considered "poor" protein sources (e.g. only beans or only corn). However, this defect may be corrected by combining several overlapping poor sources deficient in one or another of the essential amino acids (e.g. beans plus corn), but complete when combined. How the body handles waste nitrogen is another subject, but handle it the body must.

Protein Energy and Protein Sparing

If one ingests protein and derives energy from this source, one is consuming protein for energy production and, as with carbohydrates, one gains approximately four calories from each gram of protein so utilized, about the same amount as that gained from using the same dry weight of starches or sugars. Since protein is usually more expensive to produce, the tendency throughout the world, apparently developed before these facts were understood, has been to consume starches or fats for energy and to consume protein to supply the essential amino acids for the individual's needed protein structures. By relying on the body's wonderful ability to make the requisite internal adjustments to conserve the amino acids for vital uses and to avoid wasting them in energy production, natural economy is satisfied. When carbohydrates are burned for energy production instead of amino acids being burned, we speak of their "Protein Sparing" effect. Since protein elements are a rarer and more expensive part of the ordinary diet, if they are not being used for energy production, they can be utilized for manufacturing needed protein within the body's structure. On the other hand, when used for energy production, as they may be when cost is not a factor (or in starvation) and provided they are present in excess of current needs, the economic costs of the energy thus provided will be far greater than the costs of equivalent carbohydrate energy. The extra nitrogen produced by this use may also contribute to a waste accumulation problem, although the body usually has a very elastic capacity for dealing with this type of excess. When caloric or chemical energy intake is deficient (again, as in starvation) after using available body energy stores in stored fat, the body will use the energy stored in its own protein. This survival mechanism tends to be used only as a last resort, but energy production is always given priority.

Chapter 4

Fats and Lipids, Saturation, Animal vs. Vegetable Fats, Omega Numbers, "Trans" Fats, Other Lipids, Steroid Nucleus and Cholesterol, HDLs and VHDLs, Eicosanoids, Storage Space Economy, Bariatric Surgery and Liposuction

Fats & Lipids

A more correct and inclusive name for Fats is "Lipids," particularly when discussing the body's chemistry, but the more commonly used name is "Fats". Although the chemical class naming is based on simple solubility characteristics, fats can be very complex molecules. The basic chemical structure of most triglycerides or complete fat molecules lies in the attachment of three linear carbon chains (called "fatty acids") to the simple three carbon tri-alcohol (Glycerol, *Figs. 1.8* and *4.1a*). Individual fatty acids become side chains and are attached to the

Glycerol molecule via each of the glycerol molecule's alcohols (-OH) through the carbonic acid terminus at one end of each fatty acid chain. Although very weak, each fatty acid chain does contain an acidic terminal at one end and therefore is properly called an acid. These molecular components of the larger fat molecule, although very weak, consequently are all called "Fatty Acids". The general formula for the Fatty Acids is seen in *Fig. 4.1b.*

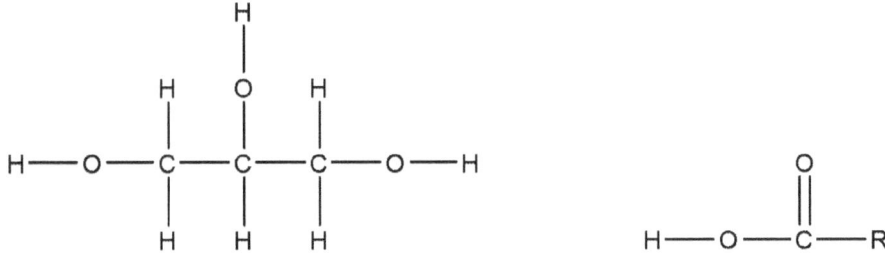

Figure 4.1a Glycerol

Figure 4.1b Generic formula for Fatty Acids
(R = Any Carbon Chain)

In that figure and elsewhere "R" can represent a single carbon atom or more complex structures. Most fatty acids contain at least 8, or a higher, usually an even number, of linearly linked, or "chained," carbon atoms. The number in most fatty acids is usually even, probably because of the method by which the they are thought to be made. This may be from various two-carbon building blocks. Fatty acids are usually "oily" and are found throughout both the vegetable and animal kingdoms; sometimes as liquids. Animal oils tend to be firmer and "saturated" (i.e. all single bonds between the several carbon atoms in each chain; also-called fully hydrogenated), while vegetable oils tend to be "unsaturated," with single or multiple double bonds (each double bonded carbon atom lacking one Hydrogen atom) and therefore having a higher potential, or stored energy (See Chapter 1 and the next paragraph). The complete fat molecule looks like:

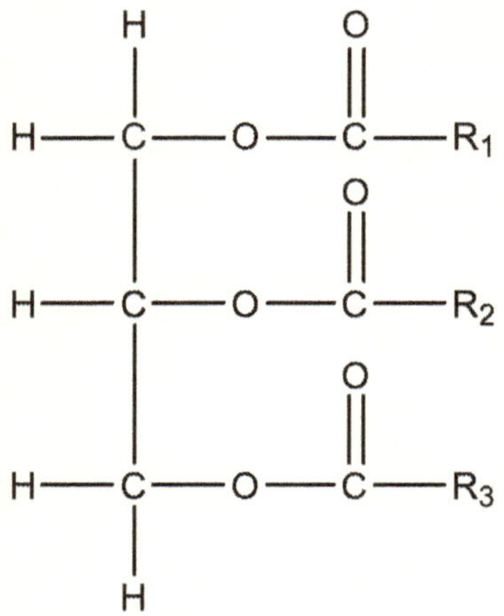

Figure 4.2 A Complete Fat Molecule
Where $C_3H_5O_3$= Glycerol portion, and $R_{1, 2 \& 3}$ = various Fatty Acid portions

All three side chains may be of the same fatty acid (i.e. $R_1=R_2=R_3$).

Saturation

Among the various side chain fatty acids a large variety of usually linear structures exist (mostly 8 to 20 Carbons). If at one or more of the intercarbon bonds there is a higher energy storage level and fewer Hydrogen atoms, the acids are said to be mono-or poly-unsaturated, depending on whether one or more than one double bond exists between the several adjacent carbon atoms in that particular chain. If there are no double bonds present, the acids are called "saturated" (i.e. with Hydrogen atoms). The physical characteristics (for instance their melting points and smells) vary with the length of the chains and their degree of, or lack of, complete Hydrogen atom saturation. Hydrogenation, or the process by which hydrogen atoms are artificially inserted into the incompletely saturated Fatty Acids at their double bond locations is said to "saturate" or "harden" them. They may then be called "trans fats," but this process only changes their energy or caloric value a little, and they are no longer accurately called "trans". A hardening process is used to manufacture margarine or "shortening" from various vegetable oils, which tend to be less saturated, and more liquid than animal fats. More recently, the "hardening", or hydrogenation process, has become prominent because of the correlation between higher saturated, or so-called "trans" fatty acid intake and the higher incidence of several artery diseases (see www.fda.gov re: trans fats).

In naming the fatty acids, the number of carbon atoms present is the primary determinant, and each carbon atom, usually counting upwards or away from the non-acid end, is numbered (*Fig. 4.3*). Since most animal fatty acids are of the saturated variety and a higher dietary intake of those saturated fats tends to be associated with diseases due to arterial hardening, it has been postulated that a lower intake and consumption of saturated fats might decrease the incidence of arterial hardening and its complications. It has been demonstrated that higher levels of blood cholesterol occur with higher saturated fat diets.

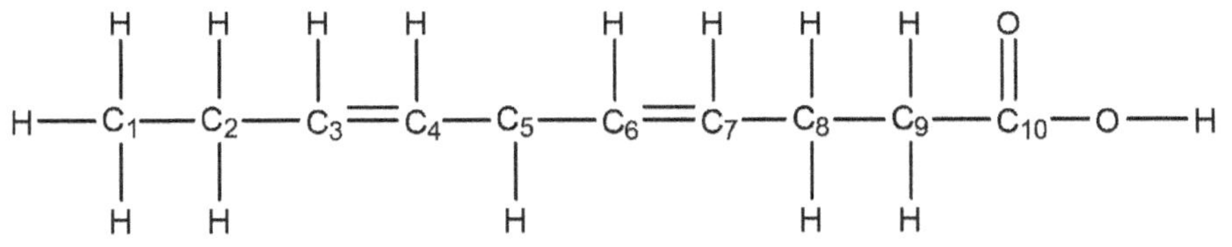

Figure 4.3 Ten Carbon Fatty Acid with Omega Number 3. Unsaturated at 3 and 6

Animal vs. Vegetable Fats and Omega Numbers (Trans Fats)

Fats and fatty oils derived from vegetable or cold fish sources tend to be less saturated. That can be changed by the Hydrogenation or "hardening" process (e.g. canned vegetable cooking fat or margarine; the so-called "trans fats"). Some food processing uses these artificially "hardened" vegetable fatty acids. Because those foods have been implicated in the development of diseases due to arterial plaques, they are considered less desirable, or heart unhealthy. This is the thinking behind the recent Federal requirement for "trans fats" labeling. Of course, until we revise our thinking about the benefits of deep fat frying (e.g. cooking donuts or french fries by immersion in boiling animal or "hardened" vegetable oil) or of having gobs of margarine on our bread, breakfast bagel, or toast, we are doomed to continue to suffer the effects of hard arteries, much brought about by our ignoring this information. Fish oil has developed an enviable reputation as "unsaturated," since most cold blooded fish oils have at least one double intercarbon bond. Contrary to the usual numbering system, the location of the bond nearest to the chain end opposite the acid end is used to describe the location of the double bonds in these molecules, and they are called "omega oils". Many nut oils have similar configurations. Therefore 3-, 6-, or 9-omega oils (common in fish and some vegetable oils) are considered more "healthful". Each omega number indicates the location of the first double bond, counting Carbon atoms upwards from the non-acid end (see *Fig. 4.3*). Conjecture, based on observations, supports this reputation.

"Trans Fats"

With the recent development of a correlation between what have been called "trans fats" and arterial disease, it becomes important to try first to understand what "trans fats" really are. Looking back to the discussion on isomerism (End of Chapter 1), in combination with the above discussion on "omega numbers", it is apparent that the relatively rigid double bond between adjacent Carbon atoms in the Fatty Acids may exist with the single Hydrogen atoms either on the same (cis) or opposite (trans) sides of the carbon chain (see *Fig. 4.4a,b* for diagrammatic representation.).

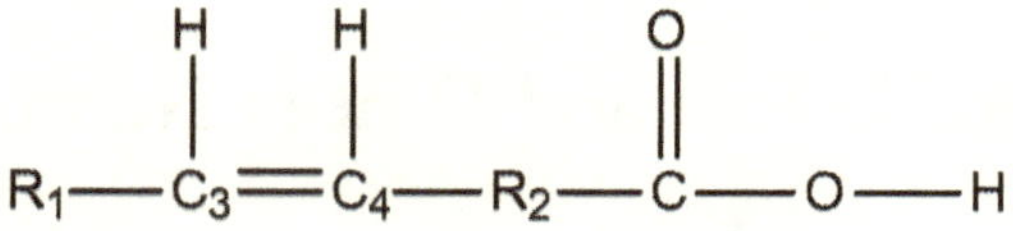

$$R_1 - C_3 = C_4 - R_2 - C - O - H$$

Figure 4.4a "Cis" configuration, (Refer to *Fig. 4.3*) R_1 & R_2 = Different Carbon Chains

$$R_1 - C_3 = C_4 - R_2 - C - O - H$$

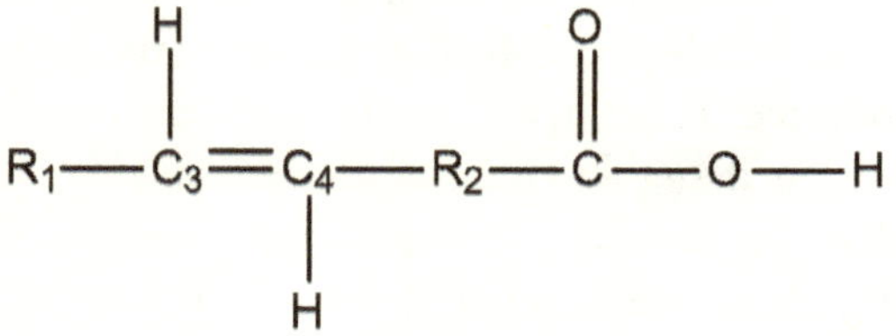

Figure 4.4b "Trans" configuration, R_1 & R_2 = Different Carbon Chains, same as Fig. 4.4a

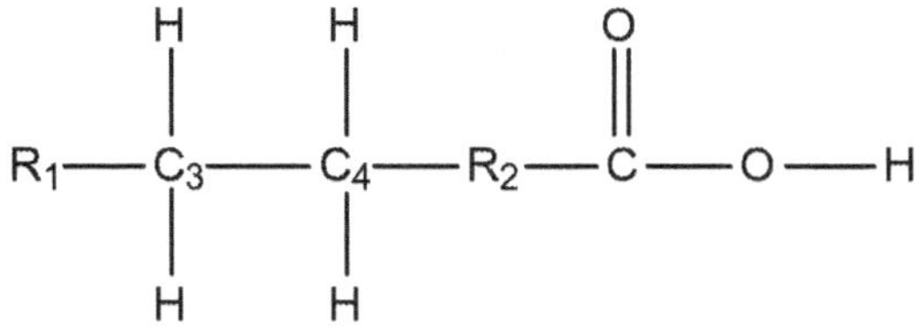

Figure 4.4c Saturated C3 to C4 Bond, (neither "Cis" nor "Trans"), R1&R2 = Different Carbon Chains, same as Fig. 4.4a & Fig. 4.4b.

Most vegetable and cold fish unsaturated fatty acids are found to be in the "cis" configuration. When the hydrogenation process is carried out to completion, all the double bonds become saturated so that the terms "cis" and "trans" no longer apply (*Fig. 4.4c*). However, if the process is incomplete (as it frequently is), some of the so-called saturated fats may not be saturated, but the results of the "hardening" process are referred to as "trans" fats, primarily considering the source of the fat. Thus, in reality, "trans fats" is a misnomer, but an understandable short-cut to the likely source designation (also "heart unhealthy" characteristics). Although it has yet to be demonstrated that reducing saturated (or formerly "trans") fat intake will actually reduce hard artery diseases, it does make good sense to make that assumption. FDA label rules require processed foods to carry this information after 1Jan2006.

Other Lipids

In some fatty molecules, one or two atoms of sulfur or phosphorous, usually a portion of an amino acid, are made a part of a larger structure. Other lipids may be formed by inclusion of one or more other amino acids in their molecular structure, and still others by inclusion of other molecules. These various fatty substances fall into the larger group called "other lipids". There are many other types of molecules that are considered fatty substances, primarily because of their solubility characteristics. These very complex molecules are included among the lipids, although some, like cholesterol, are composed solely of Oxygen, Carbon, and Hydrogen and therefore, except for solubility characteristics, really qualify as carbohydrates. Complex lipids are found throughout the body, particularly in the Central Nervous System (CNS: brain and spinal cord) where they are usually found with one or more phosphorous atoms attached. These compounds are called "phospholipids". Probably because of their unique abilities as electrical insulators, as well as their ability to be water soluble on one side of the molecule and fat soluble on the other, lipids are also an important part of most cell membranes and intracellular organelles and are found in every cell throughout the entire body. They are also the body's main means of transporting fatty substances from one place to another within the body via the blood serum. Other molecules, because of their components, may be formed from lipids and starches and are therefore called "glycolipids". Molecules containing Phosphorus and lipids are called "phospholipids" etc.

Essential Fats

Several of the Fatty Acids have been found to be essential to growing children. None of them are actually complete Fats. They are listed here and in Chapter 8 (see Figs. 4.5 & 8.2):

Linoleic Acid: $C_{18}H_{30}O_2$ (two double bonds)
alpha Linolenic Acid: $C_{18}H_{30}O_2$ (three double bonds)
Arachidonic Acid: $C_{20}H_{32}O_2$ (four double bonds)

Figure 4.5 "Essential" Fatty Acids

Steroid Nucleus & Cholesterols

Another important lipid molecule (*Figs. 1.13* and *4.6a*) is called the steroid nucleus. This nucleus is the basic structure for many biologically important molecules, particularly hormones. Hormones are chemical messengers sent from one area of the body to another usually via the blood stream (see the part of Chapter 16 on Hormones). Many hormones have a steroid nucleus as their basic structure. Cholesterol (*Fig. 4.6b*) is also built on this nucleus. Among other places in which Cholesterol may be found are in arterial plaques, sometimes in the form of crystals, or even calcified. Of course, it is also found in relatively high concentrations in egg yolks and organ meats. It's intake is probably best avoided, but since Cholesterol can be manufactured by the body anyway, it will be produced if the body needs it. Nevertheless, it remains a very important molecule nutritionally and physiologically, although not classified as "essential" in the diet (since the body can manufacture it if a need is sensed). From the diagram (*Fig 4.6b*), it is apparent why the Cholesterol molecule is classified with the carbohydrates, although its solubility allows it to be considered with the lipids.

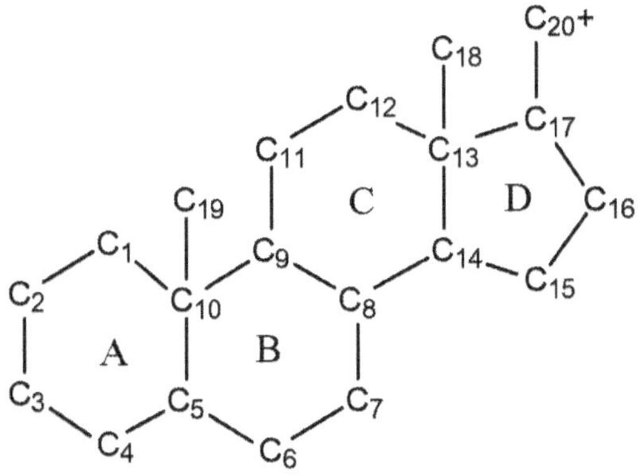

Figure 4.6a Steroid Nucleus: Ring & Carbon Atom Numerization, Hydrogen atoms understood. An Oxygen atom may be and usually is attached somewhere.

Here are some examples of varieties of prominent steroid nucleus based chemicals, where the additional part of the molecule looks like:

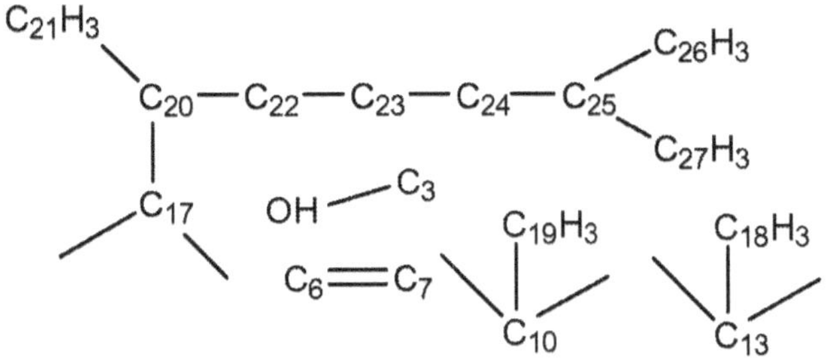

Figure 4.6b Cholesterol (The inter-Carbon bond between Carbon numbers 6 & 7 is unsaturated, most Hydrogen atoms are understood.)

Here are some other frequently encountered modifications of the Steroid Nucleus (see *Figure 4.6a* for orientation):

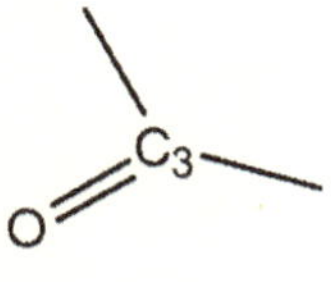

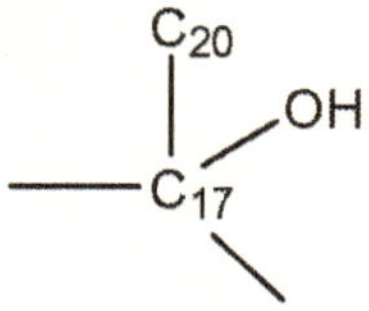

Figure 4.7a 3-Keto-   *Figure 4.7b* 17-Hydroxy-(Again, most Hydrogen atoms understood.)

Cholesterol Measurement

Most of the cholesterol circulating in fasting human blood is complexed with proteins and the complexes are called "Lipoproteins". A part of many blood tests is the determination of Total Cholesterol, Low Density Cholesterol, High Density Cholesterol, and Triglycerides. When Lipid profiles are reported, the actually measured components, the total cholesterol, the high density lipoprotein (HDL) and the triglycerides are used to calculate the low density lipoprotein (LDL). Other minor fractions are included in the above numbers and the precision and variables have been extensively considered (Reference: The National Cholesterol Education Program within the National Institutes of Health). Actually, the Lipids found in Blood are the body's way of moving fatty substances around the body, or "transporting" them, within the blood stream as well as reflecting the general "fat health" of the individual.

LDL (Low Density, or Bad) Lipids and HDL (High Density, or Good) Lipids

Lipids in the blood are categorized as "good" or "bad" depending on whether their solutions migrate more swiftly (low density, or bad) or more slowly (high density, or good) in an electric field or other, comparable measurements of density. Both are composed of the Cholesterol molecule complexed with protein, although LDLs and HDLs are frequently confused with that molecule. A high blood level of LDLs has been found to be associated with increased heart attack mortality. Therefore, concepts of "Good" or "Bad" have been attached to these lipid levels because of the correlations found between their blood levels and their association with the complications of arterial hardening in several large studies, particularly in arteries supplying the heart muscle ("heart attacks") or the brain ("strokes"). The levels of these lipids measured in the blood are a good reflection of what's actually happening in the body. There also is quite good evidence demonstrating a correlation between exercise level, unsaturated fat food intake and blood lipid composition, although the exact desirable ranges of each are unknown. Although reasonably suspected, proof that the lipid levels are truly "good" or "bad" lacks agreement, but at least from anecdotal evidence, it is probably true. (For instance, during World War II, when starving Norwegians had relatively lipid poor diets, their heart attack rate dropped. Of course, they were also eating more cold fish then.)

Eicosanoids

Another class of long chain lipid molecules consists of several structures that participate intimately in multiple chemical reactions within the body. Given the general name eicosanoids (twenty and greater carbon chain structures), they represent not only the few "essential" fatty acids, but also several of the incompletely understood, but vital local hormones like the prostaglandins. A description of the intimate chemical changes that take place, both in the building up and the using of the various lipids, is extremely complex and far beyond our compass, but worth considering in passing. However, fortunately or unfortunately, most of these various types of fat are nature's way of making, capturing, and storing potential or chemical energy. That also means that they are very efficient foods.

Space Conservation and Food Energy

Efficient space utilization requires that the potential energy of any fat or fatty acid not immediately needed by the body be stored in as small a volume of space as possible. Later, when needed, the body is able to produce the previously stored energy when the fat is broken down or "mobilized" by the body (9 Calories for each gram of fat so used). In comparison, proteins and starches, each of which can be used in cases of starvation, produce only 4 Calories per gram (See Chapters 2, 3, and 6). Consequently, when not immediately used or burned, proteins and starches are a less efficient space energy storage method for the body. We know that a gram of dry potato (almost pure starch) or a gram of lean, dry meat (almost pure muscle and, hence, protein) or egg white (pure albumin) will produce considerably less (4/9) energy than will a gram of pure fat (e.g. butter) when metabolized. Since our dietary preparation habits rely on the cooking and consuming of numerous fats (e.g. various oils, butter, whole eggs, fatty or "well marbled" meats) as well as the ingestion of the more complex fat containing materials, like organs, we of Western civilizations become used to, and seem to develop a preference for, a diet containing many of these fatty items. Likewise, if our bodies are presented with more potential chemical energy than we currently require, in its infinite wisdom (very likely a survival characteristic selected for in our Darwinian background), our bodies, instead of rejecting the immediately unneeded energy, will store it for later use.

Energy Storage

The most architecturally efficient way of accomplishing energy storage is by manufacturing fat that is then deposited in special cells dedicated to that purpose. In this manner, currently unneeded potential caloric energy is retained. Since fat cells occur throughout the body, the specific storage location, or the one to which any excess energy to be stored will be directed, is presently unknown, but some think they can control this. Again, many claims in this area are not only unsubstantiated, but unsubstantionable. That has never deterred those profiting from an unsustantiable claim. Although there has been a suggestion that the number of fat cells in the body determines the amount of energy stored and its distribution, the plain fact is that energy intake beyond the immediate needs of any organism results in the production and through many intermediate steps, the storage, of fat.

Although the distribution of fat cell storage in any specific location might look like greater storage in one location over another, this is a very difficult proposition to prove. Given the facts that potential fat storage cells exist throughout the entire body, and that some fat can be found, even in starving individuals, excess energy or fat storage location can be almost anywhere. It does appear true that new fat cells can form during early childhood growth periods, but apparently not later.

Certain locations tend to be composed of stable fat amounts (e.g. the brain); others seem to be readily expandable (e.g. the subcutaneous, buttock and abdominal storage sites). Whether or not specific subcutaneous locations (e.g. arms, abdomens, buttocks, and lateral thighs) are selective storage loci is actually unknown, probably unknowable, and likely moot. Since an excess of energy expenditure over energy consumption will result in a diminution of fat throughout the entire body in time, when it happens, this diminution may not necessarily occur uniformly throughout the body, and may not be simultaneous. But the absolute requirement for lowering caloric intake to achieve negative energy balance is an integral and the first part of any weight reduction program. In any case, people who complain about predelicted fat storage, tend to reduce these "predelicted" sites when their excessive fat stores are truly reduced. Too often ignored in many weight loss programs, is the additional absolutely essential requirement for permanent life-style change.

Bariatric Surgery and Liposuction

In an effort to lower the amount of potential energy absorbed from various foods presented to the body, several mechanical methods have been developed by which the body is "fooled" into believing that it has taken in enough food. Some of these methods rely on bypassing a variable length of the absorbing surface of the inner lining of the intestine (mucosa), some by limiting the size of the gastric pouch, with or without an intestinal bypass to convince the subject that the entire stomach is full. Which method works best, or presents the least long-or short-term danger, has yet to be determined.

Likewise, individual fat cells can be removed by the process called "Liposuction," with some temporary reduction locally in the individual's fat storage capacity at the site of the liposuction. However, unless a truly negative caloric balance is achieved, removing cells with fat storage capacity has yet to be established as a permanent way to eliminate unwanted bulges. Again, life-style changes also must be adopted for permanent results.

Chapter 5

Enzymes, Coenzymes, Vitamins, Ergs, Endoergic and Exoergic Reactions, Energy Nomenclature, "Work", Work Beyond Basal

Enzymes and Coenzymes

Virtually every chemical reaction that takes place within the body relies on the presence of other chemical substances to facilitate the reaction. These substances, called enzymes, must be present where and when they are needed, or the reactions will not proceed. In some reactions, another molecule, called a coenzyme, must also be present in addition to the enzyme for that particular reaction to proceed. Should the enzyme function be somehow blocked, that specific reaction and subsequent reactions that depend on the product of the first reaction will not take place. So essential are these enzymes and coenzymes, that their absence or even a partial interference with some of their functions can cause almost instant cessation of some immediately vital processes and death. Most enzymes are protein molecules with very complex structures, although some have a relatively simple configuration.

Enzymes and coenzymes are characterized not only by their necessary presence but also by the fact that they are not consumed in the reactions in which they participate. In a discussion of nutritional processes, it is important to realize that although we have mentioned several reactions as proceeding from one point to the next, there can be and usually are many intermediate steps, known more intimately to the biochemists. Various enzymes, which are usually made up locally by specialized body cells, are frequently necessary for these reactions to proceed from one intermediate stage to the next. Although some enzymes and coenzymes are rather simple in chemical configuration, most are forbiddingly complex. No matter how vital they are to the many chemical reactions in which they participate, by definition, enzymes are not consumed in the reactions in which they participate and are restored to their original form after fulfilling their functions.

Vitamins

Most vitamins are actually enzymes, functioning as chemical process facilitators. Although they can be lost or wasted after being used, eventually, they need to be replaced. It is for this reason that they become a mandatory part of the nutritional program. Consequently, a vitamin supply is essential and they all must be supplied in a useful form. The body can and does make minor changes in some pre-vitamin structures enabling the absorbed vitamin pre-form to be used after it has been changed into a usable configuration. More on vitamins can be found in Chapter 7.

Ergs, Endoergic, and Exoergic Reactions

An "erg" is a tiny unit of energy or work described as a centimeter-gram-second, or the amount of energy required to lift a gram of weight at sea level one centimeter in one second. Ergs provide a convenient way to indicate or measure whether a chemical reaction requires energy before it can go forward (endoergic or endothermic), or actually produces or releases energy (exoergic or exothermic). Since most of the food we consume has energy stored within it as "potential energy", as the various reactions needed for ongoing life proceed in the body, the reactions can ultimately result in either the usual production of energy (exoergic), or the less common consumption of energy (endoergic), without actually producing or requiring what we commonly understand to be work or heat. If one thinks of the body as a wondrous chemical machine, the actual work performed in simply staying alive, like the heart's work in pumping blood, or the intestine's work in moving the food along the intestinal canal, or even the simple process of keeping each cell alive requires "work" or energy expenditure of some sort. All of this "work" is endoergic. This is called the basal, minimal work or calorie consumption required that must go on continually to simply stay alive.

Energy Nomenclature

Although the energy within the various foods we consume exists there in potential form, those who are called "thermo-chemists" prefer to consider the so-called "buried" or potential energy within any food in caloric or "thermal" terms. The usefulness of this preference can be seen when one attempts to compare the potential or buried potential energy within several different foods and food groups. Although this comparison is rough, the general principles are reliable, and the varying inter-group comparisons, e.g. the Specific Dynamic Action, or SDA, of the several food groups are best ignored in menu planning and in evaluating dietary advice. When one contemplates comparing the intake of carbohydrates or proteins to fats, the nine to four ratio is the important fact to be considered. This is especially true when contemplating a large weight loss.

"Work" and Work Beyond Basal

The extra work of exercise, moving about, or of what we commonly understand to be "work" or job requirements needs even more energy expenditure in addition to those basal, resting, metabolic requirements. Since the body's method of energy storage is relatively efficient, and it's ability to retrieve energy from that previously stored is also efficient, most people are able to ignore the intimate details of the potential energy or the work storage process and pay attention only to the result, measured in body weight. Even though the energy stored can be considered "potential," it is real and really there in stored form. Enzymatic participation is usually necessary both to accomplish the storage and to release the stored potential energy. Energy production and use are discussed in greater detail in Chapter 7, and the BMR or Basal Metabolic Rate in Chapter 6.

Chapter 6

Caloric Values, Kilocalories, Calories vs. Food Weight, Basal Metabolic Rate (BMR) and "Work", Work beyond Basal, Energy Interchangeability and Consumption, Energy Related Definitions: METS, Joules, Work, Ergs, and Dynes

Calories

A calorie is a physical unit of energy and is defined as the amount of heat required to elevate the temperature of a cubic centimeter of pure water from 15 to 16 degrees Centigrade. Although this definition refers only to the tiny quantity of physical heat (or molecular motion) required to raise a milliliter of water one degree Centigrade, the energy represented can either exist as real, present energy in the form of heat or as "potential" energy, stored within the chemical structures of various foods for subsequent release and use.

Kilocalories

When Nutritionists speak of food Calories, they are actually talking about Kilocalories or so much "potential" energy, stored within various foods. A Kilocalorie is one thousand calories. As nutritionists do, we will use that convention, usually indicating it with a capital "C" (see Carbohydrate Energy in Chapter 2).

Since heat is actual thermal energy or molecular motion, a food Calorie is a measure of the amount of heat energy a specific amount of food might produce, but is presently being stored chemically within the food; thus it is really "potential", or hidden energy. Although the body's method of obtaining the energy stored in food is quite complicated, it involves many intermediate chemical steps, most aided by enzymes. The ultimate result of food utilization is energy production.

In order to keep these concepts as simple, but as useful and understandable, as possible, various foods have been measured for their potential caloric value. It must be realized that the water and indigestible fiber, or cellulose (indigestible by humans and therefore unavailable to us) content or percentage in each food is obviously of importance in determining any food's ultimate caloric value (i.e. how dilute the calories are) as opposed to the weight of the food to be consumed. All Carbohydrates, including table sugar (Chapter 2), and Proteins (Chapter 3), produce about four Calories per dry gram when completely utilized. Fats (Chapter 4) produce nine. Ethanol (Chapter 2) is the main exception to all three, producing seven Calories per gram. These numbers are immutable, and the facts implied are inescapable.

Thus, a dry gram of plain potato (almost pure starch) or a dry gram of muscle or egg white (almost pure protein) will contain four Calories and simple multiplication will enable anyone to calculate the energy potential by knowing how much of the caloric value (dry weight times available Calories) to be consumed and presented to the body (exclusive of water or indigestible fiber) is actually present. For example, simple table sugar provides four Calories per gram, is usually dry, and is usually completely absorbed, so that its caloric value can be readily computed from the weight ingested.

Calories vs. Food Weight

Complications arise when trying to estimate the water or fiber (non-caloric) content of each foodstuff, in addition to the fat content of any particular food.

The non-calorie bearing parts of each food, like water, have no impact on the energy supply. Therefore humanly unusable parts of the diet, like the various fibers or celluloses, do contain calories, but not for humans. Because they contribute to the food weight and character, they are a meaningful part of any restricted diet, but because the buried, or potential, calories are inaccessible to humans, the cellulose content can be ignored. Yet in order to continue to exist, our bodies, or chemical machines if you will, even when doing nothing but growing older, have an ongoing daily requirement for energy. If one thinks of the body as a machine deriving its fuel chemically, the work performed in simply staying alive, even the simple process of keeping each cell alive, requires "work", or caloric energy expenditure of some sort. Foods with parts inaccessible for human use, like the various "fibers", are devoid of meaningful calories and might just as well be water. This is the true meaning of the phrase "empty calories". Digestible fat energy is an entirely different story. Because the gross weight of a food portion only begins to indicate the true caloric value or potential energy available in that amount of food, someone contemplating a reduced energy intake needs to take pains to find the actual caloric value to be consumed. Also, there are a few foods, such as lettuce, or celery that require more mechanical energy to eat and potential energy to digest than they supply in food or caloric value. These few foods may be considered truly calorically negative, or endoergic.

Basal Metabolic Rate (BMR) and "Work"

The basic work being done all the time by our bodies is fundamental to ongoing life and is the work measured in the resting basal metabolic rate, or "BMR". In the performance of this resting work, calories are used. Since this requirement must be met while sustaining life, it represents a sort of caloric floor; different for every individual. The BMR usually requires in the neighborhood of 1400 to 1800 Calories/day, but can vary for any individual.

Work Beyond Basal

The extra energy used by what we commonly understand to be "work," or job requirements, calls for caloric expenditure above and beyond the basal metabolic needs. (This subject also was mentioned in Chapter 5.) When more than basal work requirements are demanded, such as when we exercise or shiver to keep warm, more work is being done, and consequently, more Calories are being burned to accomplish this work. Non-job related or "recreational" exercise falls into this "extra use" category.

The total daily energy requirement is not fixed, but varies not only with the individual's size, sex, and age, but also with his or her ongoing extra requirement. It can be either higher or lower, occasionally much higher or much lower. Since the body can be fooled (hormonally) into behaving as if the basal requirement is higher than it needs to be, some excess caloric expenditure can be falsely achieved artificially by raising the body's metabolic thermostat, or demand, for caloric expenditure. But the ultimate health impairment cost paid for artificial caloric burning achieved by hormonally fooling the body in this manner is unacceptably high.

Illness, in the form of fever or excessive thyroid activity can create abnormal thermal behavior. When illness causes fever, or the body's response to an illness results in fever and a higher metabolic rate, this and the other body responses are suspected to be helpful in combating, or at least in diagnosing, the illness. A moderate fever is accepted as a helpful part of the body's response in the context of normal healing. Whether this is actually true, of course, is not known, but it is known that fever itself can become excessive at times, and when too high can ultimately become destructive.

Energy Interchangeability

We have seen that chemical energy, stored as potential energy within food, is derived from the various foods we eat. We have also seen that this potential energy can be converted from those foods and approximately how much potential energy is derived from each class of food. Since the body's method of energy storage is so efficient, and since the body's ability to retrieve energy from its store is also efficient, those of us not burdened with excess fat are able to ignore the intimate details of the energy (work potential) storage processes and pay attention only to the ultimate result, or body weight. We now need to understand that this potential energy can be traded back and forth between the various storage locations within our bodies, usually by enzyme facilitated reactions. This energy can also be used to satisfy ongoing energy requirements within each living cell. If the body's total daily requirement is raised above the basal need by activity, then more energy will be needed to support this activity. This is the thinking underlying the advocacy of exercise in weight reduction programs. It is also why lumberjacks, said to be among the highest of Calorie using workers, probably burn over 5,000 Calories a day.

Consuming high protein foods (at 4 Calories/Gm) also feels like more food being eaten, primarily because of slower Gastric emptying (considered in Chapter 13). However, the higher protein diets which use this phenomenon tend to be much more expensive. On the other hand, less expensive high carbohydrate diets can be used for almost all energy needs, and carbohydrates used for this purpose are lauded as "protein sparing", because very little protein is being used for energy production and the more expensive amino acids in the proteins are thus available for other, more pressing body purposes (considered under Protein Sparing in Chapter 3). Since both carbohydrates and proteins provide about four calories per each gram of dry food absorbed and metabolized, they can be considered calorically equivalent. Fats or the other molecules in the lipid category (Chapter 4) not only delay Gastric emptying, but supply nine calories per gram, and thus, are much higher (9/4ths) in stored potential chemical energy. When considering the caloric value of various foods, it is important to understand that the water content and the indigestible fiber content of each food have no effect on the food's caloric impact.

The healthy human body is able to interconvert most caloric energy, setting it's own priorities. The continuation of life's activities, in the form of basal metabolism, apparently has the highest metabolic priority. The fasting or starving individual will utilize the available energy stored in most of the individual's fat cells first, then attack other potential energy stores, such as muscle. However, when ongoing nutritional needs are not being met by intake, in its innate wisdom, the body first uses energy stored in Liver starch or glycogen, and then the energy available in fat. When those sources are depleted it attacks and breaks down muscle and other amino acid stores. (One needs only to think of pictures of the Holocaust victims or persons suffering from anorexia to visualize the results of starvation.)

Energy Consumption

There is some information available to guide individuals seeking to increase their caloric use or food burning with exercise. As an example, we present data extracted from a tome on nutrition here:

Activity	60 Kg female	80 Kg male
Sitting Quietly	1.2 Cal/hr.	1. 7 Cal/hr.
Hard Swimming	9 Cal/hr.	12 Cal/hr.
Power Walking	4.7 Cal/hr.	6.4 Cal/hr.

Figure 6.1 Approximate Energy Consumption Table, or Calories Burned per minute, Extracted from: Appendix, Krause's: Food, Nutrition and Diet Therapy, 9th Edition, Saunders

Energy Related Definitions: Joules, METS, Work, Ergs, and Dynes

METS is an abbreviation for "Metabolic Equivalent," defined in Steadman's Medical Dictionary (26th Ed.) as "the oxygen cost of energy expenditure (production) measured at supine rest, or 1MET = 3.5ml consumed O_2 per Kg of body weight per minute." In other words a basal MET is the amount of energy (i.e. Calories) one requires or burns simply to stay alive and awake per minute, based on, and varying with, the individual's weight. But an extra MET is a useful measure of the effect of any particular exercise (also noting it's duration). Moreover, we know that the basic metabolism required to keep a fat storage cell alive for a minute is a lot less than that required for an active cell (Liver cell, for instance). Consequently, a MET will vary not only with the basic weight of the subject and the subject's percentage of fat, but also the physical work being done by the individual, and the total being used by each cell in each person.

Elsewhere, we have mentioned the difficulty of determining the "best" or ideal weight (for BMI and ideal weight discussion see Chapter 7), and the MET is another example of how the body fat percentage complicates the picture. On the other hand, METS are extensively used to give some approximation of effort being expended by various activities, e.g. 3 to 5 METs for light work; more than 9 METs for heavy work (Steadman, again). METs are used as a good general guide to the amount of exercise an individual is performing at any particular time.

JOULES. A Joule is the amount of force required to accelerate one Kilogram one Meter per second per second and is equal to 100,000 dynes (Webster). A dyne is the amount of force required to accelerate one Gram one Centimeter per Second per Second. Joules are hardly ever encountered in nutritional discussions.

WORK is defined as the transfer of energy or heat or molecular motion from one physical system (e.g. a shovel, a flame or sunlight) to another (e.g. a rock, a chemical or a plant), or the use of a muscle contraction to produce a result.

ERG. A unit of energy or work needed to raise one Gram one Centimeter in one Second. 1 Erg=1 Centimeter Gram Second, obviously very small.

DYNE. The force or power needed to accelerate one Gram of mass one Centimeter per Second per Second. 1 Dyne=1 Gram per Second per Second, like-wise tiny.

Chapter 7

Standards and Storage, Water, RDAs, Minerals and Vitamins, Energy and Calories-ongoing Requirements plus, Sensing Needs, Standard Height and Weight Tables, BMI, BMI Problems, Morbid Obesity

Standards and Storage

Every body has a number of requirements that must be met in order to survive and function normally, like air, shelter, rest, food, and water. For completeness and to place some of these requirements in nutritional perspective we mention several of them in this Chapter.

Water

Since water is not an atomic element, but a not-so-simple molecule made up of two elements *(Fig. 1.1a)*, it cannot be classified among the necessary elements. However, there are many vital molecules, including water. All vital substances should be taken in on an almost daily basis.

Although the human minimum volume intake of needed water is probably around a liter a day, the amount actually required is determined by the ability of the Kidneys to concentrate waste products for elimination. A desirable minimal urine output of about 30 ml/hr or 720 ml/24hrs is considered adequate if the Kidneys are functioning normally. Of course, if the Kidneys are concentrating wastes less efficiently, the urine output needs to be higher. Some water is also a by-product of energy production from various food molecules so the body gains water from the food breakdown processes, but it is usually not enough to satisfy the daily requirement. Since our bodies can only minimally store it, we should have some form of real water on an almost daily basis to maintain that output.

Foods & Recommended Daily Allowance (RDA)

Because various nutriments are considered "essential," and since the Food and Nutrition Board of the United States National Academy of Sciences-National Research Council has issued a Table that states the "average daily intake" or "Recommended Dietary Allowances" of several macronutrients for several classes of people per day, we abstract it here:

Nutrient:	Adult Women:	Adult Men:
Digestible Carbohydrate	130 Grams/day	130 Grams/day
Fiber	26 Grams/day	38 Grams/day
Total Fat	20-35 Grams/day	20-35 Grams/day
Total Protein +	46 Grams/day	56 Grams/day

Figure 7.1 Table of Food Recommended Daily Allowances (RDA)
+Must include the "indispensable" (i.e. "essential") Amino Acids (Chapter 3)

Several other nutrients are omitted from the Table because their requirements are "less well defined." These average daily recommendations are considered min-imal, although they are safe-sided estimates. The RDA Table also recommends a quantity of protein for various weights, but contains no recommendation of protein type, nor of ideal bodyweight.

Minerals & Vitamins

Since there are minimal recommendations for several of the minerals and vitamins, these can be used in designing one's own food intake. Although a daily intake is convenient for quantitating the essentials, an adequate total weekly intake would be most unlikely to result in any dietary harm, provided the essentials are presented for the body to use in sufficient quantity. With the recent advent of meaningful food labels it has become possible to ensure an adequate intake, if not on a daily basis, at least weekly. For the unique case of Sodium, the reader is referred to the discussion of that atom in Chapter 20.

Element & Symbol	Women, RDA*	Men, RDA*	UL*
Calcium, Ca	1,200 mg/d	1,200 mg/d	2,500 mg/d
Copper, Cu	900 ug/d	900 ug/d	10,000 ug/d
Fluorine, F	3 ug/d	4 ug/d	10 ug/d
Iodine, I	150 ug/d	150 ug/d	1,100 ug/d
Iron, Fe	8-18 mg/d	8 mg/d	45 mg/d
Magnesium, Mg	320 mg/d	420 mg/d	350/450 mg/d
Molybdenum, Mo	45 ug/d	45 ug/d	2,000 ug/d
Phosphorus, P	700 mg/d	700 mg/d	4,000 mg/d
Selenium, Se	55 ug/d	55 ug/d	400 ug/d
Zinc, Zn	8 mg/d	11 mg/d	49 mg/d

Figure 7.2 Table of Minerals (*RDA=Recommended Dietary Allowances; UL=Upper Safe Daily Limit. Omitted: Arsenic, Boron, Chromium, Manganese, Nickel, Silicon, Sodium, and Vanadium; mg/d=milligrams per day; ug/d=micrograms per day)

Vitamin Designation	Women, RDA*	Men, RDA*	UL*
Folate	400 ug/d	400 ug/d	1,000 ug/d
Niacin	14 mg/d	16 mg/d	35 mg/d
Riboflavin (B$_2$)	1.1 mg/d	1.3 mg/d	Not Determined
Thiamin (B$_1$)	1.1 mg/d	1.2 mg/d	Not Determined
Vitamin A #FS	700 ug/d	900 ug/d	3,000 ug/d
Vitamin B$_6$	1.3 to 1.5 mg/d	1.3 to 1.7 mg/d	100 mg/d
Cobalamin (B$_{12}$)	2.4 ug/d	2.4 ug/d	Not Determined
Vitamin C	75 mg/d	90 mg/d	2,000 mg/d
Vitamin D #FS	5 to 15 ug/d	5 to 15 ug/d	50 ug/d
Vitamin E #FS	15 mg/d	15 mg/d	1,000 mg/d
Vitamin K #FS	90 ug/d	120 ug/d	Not Determined

Figure 7.3 Table of Vitamins (#FS=Fat soluble, others Water soluble; *RDA & *UL as in *Fig 7.2*, Omitted: Biotin, Choline, and Pantothenic Acid.) Table of Recommended Dietary Vitamin Allowances, Revised 1989, Food and Nutrition Board, National Academy of Sciences-National Research Council

This means that vitamin and mineral supplements, taken a few times a week, should be adequate for most people. The brand of mineral or vitamin supplement is really irrelevant, as long as the essential ingredients are there. Food labels are required to be truthful by federal law, therefore they should be definitive (but see January '06 Consumer Reports). Growing babies, inside and outside the womb, and children after birth have higher requirements than adults on a per weight basis.

Energy and Calories, Ongoing Requirements Plus

The ongoing need for energy, potential or real, may be the least well understood requirement for continuing health. Unless the body's automatic thermostat, or metabolic rate, is set artificially or pathologically high, a normal adult body will need to burn a total of about 2,000 to 2,500 Calories a day. Of course, this varies directly with the size and activity of the individual and inversely with the age and amount of body fat. The daily energy amount used can be voluntarily increased by exerting more muscle energy or "work" (e.g. with exercise), but a short period of exercise burns off very few extra Calories. The underlying basal requirements remain. As humans grow older, their daily requirements fall, so that whereas at the age of twenty a sedentary youth might require 3,000 Cal/day as a basic need, when that same youth reaches a sedentary retirement, her daily basal need might have fallen to 1,500 Cal/day, or less, to remain in energy balance. At any age, well tolerated exercise will increase caloric expenditure, but unless the duration of the increased activity is prolonged, caloric consumption or burning will be minimal. This may account for the tendency of fat to accumulate as we grow older, unless we reduce our daily energy intake.

Sensing Needs

The body is capable of storing varying amounts of some of the essential substances. The water soluble vitamins and some of the minerals, particularly Iron in menstruating women, are almost as essential on a near daily basis as is water itself, since only very little of this atom can be stored. Moreover, the body cannot store water, nor the water soluble vitamins. Fat soluble vitamins, on the other hand, are stored in body fat. People who have large fat deposits are less likely to be depleted of the fat soluble vitamins as rapidly as thinner dieters, yet these stores, too, are also eventually expended unless replaced, making the fat soluble vitamins ultimately essential. Average daily requirements are undetermined for some of the less well understood or "trace" minerals (e.g. Chromium or Nickel), although several atoms besides Sodium and Iron are known to be vital. In some cases the body has developed mechanisms to indicate depleted requirements. Thirst, or the need for water, is a very demanding and usually a very reliable sensation. Yet our Darwinian survival characteristics have not developed to the point where we can recognize several of the other deficiencies or oversupplies. Some of the sensations, hunger for instance, are not only unreliable, but dangerous. If we pay heed to our thirst sensation, as we should, we will provide an immediately needed molecule (H_2O). If, on the other hand, we obey our hunger sensation, we will tend to supply our intestinal tracts with food our bodies may not really need, with the consequence that any excess over current needs will be taken in, and then automatically stored. Elaboration of this point, the basic thesis of this book, will be found in Chapter 18.

Standard Height & Weight Tables

Calculation of the Body Mass Index is a simple matter. The Body Mass Index is defined as the weight in Kilograms (pounds divided by 2.2) divided by the square of the height in Meters (inches multiplied by 0.0254, times itself). By using the individual's weight (in Kilograms) (then dividing that number by the height in

Meters, squared), an automatic emphasis is focused on the weight, but related to the height. Tables exist where the arithmetic has already been done after converting from the English system of measurement (pounds and inches) to Metric (Meters and kilograms). Standards have also been published purporting to correlate height, body build, sex, age, and weight. Some of these standards are simply averages obtained from a large group of people. Other tables can be obtained from insurance surveys of supposedly healthy people who have taken out life insurance. Since our society has many overweight people, those tables are probably skewed to a value much higher than they ought to be. Just as we lack a good definition of "health", so we lack a good standard definition of healthy weight.

Body Mass Index (BMI)

The BMI is a quick guide to the presence of obesity. If the calculation, when made, is found to be less than 25 it is considered normal; if over 30, overweight. A widely accepted definition of "Overweight" is a BMI between 30 and 35 in both men and women. Frank "Obesity" is over 35, and dangerous or "Morbid Obesity" is over 40, but the need to break down too much fat seems to have more to do with social or political acceptability than reality. An undernourished state is considered to exist when the BMI is less than 20, although that number is probably too high. Much below 18.5 or 19 can be a sign of poor nutrition, and much lower really dangerous.

Abbreviated (and rounded off) BMI Table, English and Metric

Height (in Meters)
"(below=Ft.&In.)

Weight in Pounds	1.47 Mtrs 4'10	1.57 Mtr 5'2	1.63 Mtr 5'4	1.68 Mtr 5'6	1.73 Mtr 5'8"	1.78 Mtr 5'10	1.83 Mtr 6'	1.98 Mtr 6'6"	Apprx. Weight in Kilos
300#	63	55	51	48	45	43	41	35	136Kg
290#	61	53	50	47	44	42	39	34	132Kg
280#	59	52	48	45	43	40	38	32	127Kg
270#	57	49	46	44	41	39	37	31	123Kg
260#	54	48	45	42	40	37	35	30	118Kg

Weight in Pounds	1.47 Mtrs 4'10	1.57 Mtr 5'2	1.63 Mtr 5'4	1.68 Mtr 5'6	1.73 Mtr 5'8"	1.78 Mtr 5'10	1.83 Mtr 6'	1.98 Mtr 6'6"	Apprx. Weight in Kilos
250#	52	46	43	40	38	36	34	29	114Kg
240#	50	44	41	39	37	35	33	28	109Kg
230#	48	42	38	37	35	33	31	27	105Kg
220#	46	40	37	36	34	32	30	26	100Kg
210#	44	38	36	34	32	30	29	24	95Kg
200#	42	37	34	32	30	29	27	23	91Kg
190#	40	35	33	31	29	27	26	22	86Kg
180#	38	33	31	29	27	26	24	21	82Kg
170#	36	31	29	27	26	24	23	20	77Kg
160#	34	29	27	26	24	23	22	19	73Kg
150#	31	27	26	24	23	22	20	17	68Kg
140#	29	26	24	23	21	20	19	16	64Kg
130#	27	24	22	21	20	19	18	15	59Kg
120#	25	22	21	19	18	17	16	14	55Kg
110#	23	20	19	18	17	16	15	13	50Kg
100#	21	18	17	16	15	14	14	11	45Kg

Figure 7.4 BMI Table, Abbreviated and Rounded

BMI Problems

At a recent American Society for Bariatric Surgery meeting in Orlando, FL the BMI alone was called "insufficient" without supplemental body habitus measurements for patient screening (American College of Surgeons "Surgery News" v1,#12,p19). Another inherent fallacy in this simple index can be best demonstrated by considering a theoretical 20 year old, 6 foot tall, 200 pound fullback in superb physical shape (see Fig. 7.5). Twenty years later, he will be as tall as he was earlier. In the unlikely case that he has gained no weight, his BMI will be the same: (200#/2.2, divided by 182.88x182.88; or 91Kg/(1.82m)^2 Both = +/-27). But even if our fullback has remained physically active, the former player's actual muscle mass likely would have declined in the intervening years. The weight difference would be made up by approximately 15 pounds (or more, if he has gained) of fat that his body has stored from various foods consumed in the interval, and converted to fat. We can estimate his playing weight muscle mass as approximately a quarter of his total weight (55 lbs.) and his later muscle mass as about three quarters of his playing muscle mass (40 lbs.). As is all too frequently the case, if our former fullback, now 40 years old, gains "only" 22 (10Kg) "harmless" pounds in the intervening years over his best or playing weight, his BMI will be (100/3.35) 29.8 or almost unchanged from his earlier BMI and within the stated limits for "normal," but his total body fat may have increased by at least 300% (i.e. from about 5 to at least 20 pounds). Some of that fat will be found in threatening cholesterol deposits in his arteries.

AGE & CONDITION	20 Years SUPERB	40 years EXCELLENT
Approximate Total Weight (100%)	200 pounds	200 pounds
Approximate Bone Weight (40%)	80 pounds	80 pounds
Approximate Organ Weight (30%)	60 pounds	60 pounds
Approximate Muscle Weight	55 pounds	40 pounds
Approximate Fat Weight	5 pounds	20 pounds

Figure 7.5 Theoretical comparison of BMIs of 20 year old athlete vs. 40 year old former athlete. Note that although the weight is the same, the fat burden has increased by 300%. (Same data as in *Fig 8.1*)

Morbid Obesity

The September 2000 Bulletin of The American College of Surgeons stated acceptance of the definition of Morbid Obesity as 100 or more pounds over "normal" body weight, but fails to define "normal," probably because it has never been agreed upon. Using the Body Mass Index (BMI) to expand the definition, the American College of Surgeons also accepts the concept that Morbid Obesity exists when the BMI exceeds 40 Kg/m^2, or greater than 35 if there are associated "significant" comorbidities, again not defining "significant". Practically speaking, anyone who's BMI is that much above any widely accepted definition of "normal" probably knows they have a problem.

PERCENTAGES of Non-institutionalized Americans, USA, 1988-94

	Healthy Weight / BMI 18.5-24.9	Overweight / BMI 25+	Obese(included in Overweight) BMI 30+
Men			
20-34 yrs	51.1	47.5	14.1
35-44 "	33.4	65.5	21.5
45-54 "	33.6	66.1	23.2
55-64 "	28.6	70.5	27.2
65-74 "	30.1	68.5	24.1
75&> "	40.9	56.5	13.2
Women, nonpregnant			
20-34 yrs	57.9	37.0	18.5
35-44 "	47.1	49.6	25.5
45-54 "	37.2	60.3	32.4
55-64 "	31.5	66.3	33.7
65-74 "	37.0	60.3	26.9
75&> "	43.0	52.3	19.2

Figure 7.6 (Abbreviated from CDC data)

What frequently fails to be noted is the essentially unknown consequences of gaining "a few harmless pounds", and the unknown harm which may be caused by them.

Chapter 8

Essentiality and Density: Water, Oxygen, Density, Specific Body Density, Changing Body Composition Effect, Carbohydrate and Fat Essentiality, Amino Acids and Complete vs. Incomplete Proteins, Elements, Minerals, Vitamins, Charlatanry

"Essentiality"

It is convenient to think of all living bodies as chemical factories. but, in addition to the individual atoms of which all substances on this earth are composed, there are a number of compounds that the chemical factories of our human bodies cannot manufacture. Every animal species is unique and a part of this uniqueness is the varying requirement for different organic chemical structures. The

Oxford Dictionary of the English Language defines "essential" as "absolutely necessary" or "indispensably requisite," and for all of the atoms and several varieties of the molecules which make up our human and many other bodies, this definition seems to fit. (On the other hand, a good definition of good health is lacking.) Because it is extremely difficult to demonstrate any particular requirement, and because there is no comparable animal model on which to perform valid dietary experiments for humans, some of the "requirements" are only best guesses. On the other hand, others are well studied and understood.

Water

The origin of life on earth as we know it may be debated without end, but what must surely be true is that every living cell on earth carries on its life processes in a watery environment. How the water gets into the cell and how it stays and is replaced are ongoing subjects of study, but that this ubiquitous substance is vital, not only for human existence, but for all living organisms on earth is beyond doubt. When considering absolute daily requirements, the water molecule cannot be overlooked. Nor can it's absolute requirement for health in humans that it be replaced as used (Chapter 7). With minimal normal storage capability, it is an essential molecule.

Oxygen

Besides water, and just as essential to every animal's metabolism (including human), is the other ingredient by which our bodies obtain energy from the fuel or food we consume. Often we speak of "burning" fuel. Understood, but frequently unmentioned in the "burning" process is the element oxygen (O_2), the second integral participant in the oxidative, or burning, process. When carbohydrates or the other foods are metabolized, or burned for energy, mostly carbon dioxide (CO_2) and water (H_2O) are produced. Although we possess no internal furnace wherein our fuels are consumed in open flames, we do have enzymatically assisted processes by which potential or chemical energy is gradually released for our use. Further, our bodies cannot store oxygen, so we are dependant on an uninterrupted supply.

Density

In order to understand the various components of body weight and how they interact it is necessary to understand the physical concept of "density". We tend to think of density as a sort of hardness, as in rocks, steel, or even hard-headedness. Actually, density of a material is usually compared with that of plain water, which is arbitrarily assigned a density of 1.0. Ocean water, with its dissolved salt, is a little more dense than fresh water, so objects which float in fresh water will float a little higher in salt water. Each element and many more complex combinations of elements are compared to water and each average specific density is determined. Since air is much lighter than water, an object containing air, such as a ship or dry sponge, will tend to float. But if a dry sponge or wood is left in water it becomes water-logged and it tends to sink, primarily because the air contained in the wood or dry sponge has been gradually displaced by water and the structure of the wood or sponge itself is heavier than water. On the other hand, oils or other fats float on water and their density is about 0.7. Similarly, fresh lung tissue, containing air like a damp sponge, tends to float like a sponge in water, but sinks as the contained air is gradually displaced by water. Muscle and bone are more dense and each has a specific density greater than 1.0, although different from each other. Both sink at once when first placed in water. Fatty tissue, being less dense, floats on water. When more than one tissue is measured, an average density can be found.

Specific Body Density

A food, or the human body, each composed of many elements, chemical molecules, or tissues of various densities, will float or sink depending on the sum of all the various amounts and densities they contain. In fact, the floating or sinking of a person in a swimming pool can vary with the extent of air in the lungs, so that a person immersed in a pool while holding a deep breath may float, whereas if the total or average body density exceeds 1.0 that same person, on exhaling the held breath and thereby reducing the volume of retained air in the lungs, may sink. Likewise, if a person contains a large volume of fatty tissue (at 0.7 specific density) their body floats a little higher or lower in the water, depending on the amount of air in the lungs. Similarly, with minimal fat and little air in the lungs, a lean person will tend to sink because their overall or average specific density is greater than 1.0.

Changing Composition Effect on Body Density

To illustrate the effects of change, we will revisit the theoretical 200 pound, 20 year old fullback in superb physical condition encountered in the last chapter. We would probably find that he had had an absolute minimum of body fat with a large and well-trained muscle mass. 20 years later, he might still be the same weight and in excellent condition, although chances are good that he would have picked up a few (so-called "harmless") pounds in the intervening years. Since his bones, brain, skin, organs, and blood would all weigh about what they did when he was twenty, those percentages of his weight would not have changed. However, his muscle mass would have become considerably less (since he would no longer be in the superb shape he was in while competing), and any weight difference would be accounted for, not by the weight lost from his muscle mass, but by the weight of the added fat he had accumulated in the interval, maintaining the same weight. Some of that difference might well have accumulated as cholesterol plaques in his arteries (*Figs. 7.5* and *8.1*), setting him up for a heart attack or stroke.

AGE & CONDITION	20 Years SUPERB	40 years EXCELLENT
Approximate Total Weight (100%)	200 pounds	200 pounds
Approximate Bone Weight (40%)	80 pounds	80 pounds
Approximate Organ Weight (30%)	60 pounds	60 pounds
Approximate Muscle Weight	55 pounds (27.5% vs.)	40 pounds (20%)
Approximate Fat Weight	5 pounds (2.5% vs.)	20 pounds (10%)

Theoretical comparison: Body Composition of 20 year old athlete vs. 40 year old former athlete with similar BMIs. Note that although the weight and BMI are the same, the fat has increased 400%

Figure 8.1 (Table reproduced from *Figure 7.5*)

Carbohydrates and "Essential" Fats

Carbohydrates, no matter how complex, consist only of Carbon (C), Hydrogen (H), and Oxygen (O) atoms. The chief exception to this classification is Cholesterol, which although chemically a carbohydrate, behaves like a fat in solubility characteristics All of the carbohydrates can be manufactured by the body (Chapter 2) through what is called "intermediate metabolism". The absence of several fatty acids (Chapter 4) from the diet results in the development of a so-called "deficiency state" which can then result in illness, particularly in a growing child. The essential fatty acids, which the body cannot manufacture, have been listed in Chapter 4 (see Fig, 4.5).

Generally, the essential fats help to form the eicosanoid compounds (thromboxane, prostaglandins, and leukotrienes). Notice that these substances are all fatty acids and not really true or complete fats at all (since they lack an attachment to glycerol). These substances participate in many of the less well studied (and more difficult to study and learn) reactions within the human body. Although no known deficiency state of these fatty acids have been detected in adults, infants do appear to be susceptible to essential fatty acid deficiencies.

Amino Acids and "Complete" Proteins vs. "Incomplete" Proteins

In a similar fashion to fats, several amino acids (see Chapter 3, Figure 3.2) are also required for health maintenance. The human body cannot manufacture them. Since there are a number of these necessary basic protein building blocks and in as much as all of them are not found in all proteins in some human diets, protein sources containing all of the essential amino acids have been called "complete" or "good" proteins. Other protein sources that lack one or another of the essential amino acids in sufficient quantity to prevent deficiency disease development when those proteins are the sole dietary source of amino acids have been called "incomplete" or "poor."

Although many inexpensive foods contain most of the various "essential" amino acids, they may lack a few. Because "complete" protein foods tend to be more expensive (and although some of the "incomplete" protein foods are considerably cheaper and more readily available) by supplementing one "poor" source to make up for the lacking ingredient, combinations of two or more overlapping "incomplete" proteins tend to be significant portions of some entirely safe human diets, particularly in the less well developed or affluent countries.

What tends often to be overlooked is the fact that the "incomplete" nature of a particular protein source can frequently be corrected either by eating protein supplements containing those missing essential amino acid(s) absent from the primary protein source or by ingesting another food containing the specific missing amino acid. This type of adjustment commonly occurs when two "poor" sources, such as beans and corn, complement each other and overlap, thereby providing the essentials missing from the primary source to provide a cheap but actually "complete" essential amino acid supply. Consequently an entirely adequate diet is achieved. Lack of a few of the "essential" amino acids in one food can be partially or completely offset by increasing the intake of some of the others, but it is wiser to consider all of the "essential" amino acids as exactly that. Apparently the pre-Columbian Inca Indians found this out. On the other hand, if enough high quality protein foods are ingested, ignoring financial cost, the "essential" amino acid requirement certainly should be met.

Elements

There are several other atoms participating in our bodies makeup, and they can most conveniently be thought of in two groups; the macro-elements and the micro-elements. Of course, we cannot create atoms, or the basic building blocks of various compounds, so that we might well consider the atoms Carbon (C), Hydrogen (H), and Oxygen (O), as essential, but this becomes more a Philosophical than a Nutritional question.

Macroelements

Macro Minerals, or macroelements, are differentiated by the adult dietary requirement of at least 100 mg/day (See *Fig. 7.2*). Among the needed macro-elements are Sodium (Na), Potassium (K), Chlorine (Cl), Phosphorous (P), Magnesium (Mg), and Calcium (Ca). Although not a true mineral, we have not mentioned water (H_2O) as an essential part of the diet (except in Chapter Seven and above), although it too is vital, not only as an intake solution base and medium for transport or circulation of nutrients within the body, but for waste elimination, both in the urine and stool. The digestion, absorption, deposition, and retention of the element Calcium, mostly in the bones, is apparently primarily under hormonal control, although other factors impact on the intake/output balance of this mineral. This is particularly true after menopause in women. Sodium is considered elsewhere (see Chapter 20).

Microelements

Several of the lesser widespread elements are an integral part of our Physiology and of our nutritional requirements. These atoms are usually called "trace" or micromineral elements, and although mostly found in all bodies in tiny quantities, they are nevertheless "vital," usually as a part of several enzymes. Among the needed microelements are Chromium (Cr), Cobalt (Co), Copper (Cu), Fluorine (F), Iodine (I), Iron (Fe), Magnesium (Mg), Selenium (Se), Zinc (Zn), and other elements as well. Sulfur (S) is also "essential" but it is a part of two of the essential amino acids and the requirement will be met by them. Many of the microelements are ingested as food contaminants, and will be missed only when the normal nutritional route is bypassed, as when total nutrition is being supplied by intravenous feeding. Although the daily amount of each essential ingredient of the diet is listed in the table, some of the numbers are given as a best guess, made with an estimated fail-safe margin. Many so-called "Super" Vitamin pills contain most of these "trace" elements, usually with maximal notice and minimal science.

Considered a "trace" element, but still "essential," is the iron atom (Fe^{++}). As an integral component of the hemoglobin molecule it is absolutely essential for normal red blood cell formation and function (i.e. it's ability to carry Oxygen). Given the obligatory Iron loss in menstrual blood, a greater requirement for Iron exists in menstruating females compared to males or post-menstruating females. This is true in spite of the body's tendency to husband its Iron stores.

Vitamins

Just as is true for a few fatty acids and some Amino Acids, other molecules exist that our human bodies cannot manufacture. Since these molecules are vital to the maintenance of a healthy state, they are vital to our well being. They have been called "vitamins," although, in essence, they are nothing more than special, required foods that our bodies cannot manufacture. Probably more hoopla has been written about these essential substances, which seem to have a unique cachet in their name, than about any other foods. Yet an understanding of their place in the nutritional scheme is very important, particularly when one is contemplating a diminished dietary intake, both of calories and the usual variety of foods. Indeed, some of the vitamins the human body needs are actually made by bacteriae within our intestinal tracts from foods presented to the intestinal bacteriae. These foods are then changed by those bacteriae, and then absorbed and used by us. Therefore, although these vitamins actually are being created within our intestines in some cases, they are not actually being made within our own internal chemical environments and by our own cells, but only within our intestines by "other" cells. (See *Fig. 7.3* for Recommended Daily Vitamin Allowances.)

Vitamin Classification

Vitamins are most conveniently considered by their water solubility, since this quality also governs which foods contain them in greater amounts, how they are absorbed (or not absorbed) and used, how and where they are stored within the body, how they are excreted, and how often they need to be replaced. For the reader's convenience, there is provided (in *Fig. 7.3*) a list of each type of vitamin within its solubility group, but we must caution that more misinformation probably exists about these particular molecules than just about any other group of nutrients. For the most part vitamins act as facilitators or enzymes in the various chemical processes within the body, but their required presence for continued health is absolute. Fortunately, in only a few cases are an excess of vitamins in the diet harmful. Parts of the normal body seem to sense and take what is needed if that substance is presented to it within the intestine (not the skin) and the unnecessary or unused excess within the intestinal tract passes out through the stool or is absorbed, then excreted in the urine. Significant vitamin utilization via the skin lacks rigorous scientific support, although it is strongly supported commercially.

Overdosage

Most of the tables give safe-sided estimates of the maximum allowable amounts of each foodstuff, although in the case of vitamin overdosage there is not usually a big toxicity problem. Where they appear to be significant is when dealing with abnormal food sources or abnormal body metabolic processing.

Charlatanry

It is unfortunate, yet true, that in the arena of "essential" foods a wide latitude exists for the making of unsupported, but not readily disprovable, claims. Caution is never misplaced here, but even one with a broad background in nutrition cannot deny many of the more outlandish claims. Demanding affirmative proof of claims seems to be the best and perhaps the only defense against them, but too often this demand is ignored. We all know how acceptable the "big lie" technique is and how the lie comes to be believed.

Since the intestinal route is the most natural one by which vitamins and other substances can be absorbed and enter the body's internal environment, there seems to be very little to be gained by choosing some other route for providing these needed compounds. This fact has not prevented pharmaceutical or cosmetic entrepreneurs from marketing vitamins in skin creams and other unproven vehicles. Further, various fruit and food suppliers advocate this or that particular vegetable or fruit as being "chock full" of one vitamin or another. It does seem to be true that the body will take whatever chemical it needs, if it is presented to it in the intestine, later discarding the unneeded.

Most vitamins are in this category, although a few can be taken in toxic amounts. An excellent example of an apparently harmless vitamin is the water soluble Ascorbic Acid (Vitamin "C"), which has been advocated as a cold preventative when taken in huge doses. Since there are about 200 viruses that can cause a cold, and since there is no reliable study that demonstrates the effectiveness of this theory, proof of effectiveness is lacking. However, since this vitamin is apparently harmless in the occasionally advocated mega-doses, there seems little to be gained in opposing this custom, only "Caveat Emptor." or in this case, "Caveat Consumor". Actually a standard (or generic) vitamin pill contains more vitamins than any particular vegetable or fruit of similar weight and those pills usually contain all a "normal" person should need on a daily basis.

Part Two

Anatomy and Physiology

Chapter 9

Introduction to Part Two: Anatomy & Physiology

We now consider the digestive processes, in the order in which the nutrients meet them, and what happens to the various food chemicals en-route. Although "chemicals" is a nasty word for some people, the basic fact is that every substance we ingest (or inhale, for that matter) is or is made up of chemicals. "Gut" is generally considered a slang word, but it is most useful anatomically when considering the entire Gastrointestinal (GI) tract, Mouth to Anus.

A brief glance at the contents provides an overview of what to expect, but although the chemical facts we have considered in this book's first part are fairly well understood, in the arena of human (and animal) gut physiology and nutrition, there are many instances of imperfect understanding and outright unknowns. Some of the digestive and psychological processes are fairly well understood. But in this area, even more than earlier, much caution needs to be exercised, lest partial information be treated as total, and the uninformed or incautious misled.

There is a large amount of information available on securing, preparing, and presenting foods. Thinking only of the daily newspaper, a significant percentage of space is devoted to encouraging the purchase of various foodstuffs. We have already alluded to the numerous books on crowded library shelves, many containing recipes. Magazines seem to be the predominant sources of advice for various ethnic and fad recipes and for eating disorders (both overeating and undereating). They also seem to have more suggestions for attractive food presentations, table settings, and accompaniments; be it music or wine, particularly around holidays. How often are we encouraged to adopt New Years Resolutions to reduce our intake after gaining several indiscreet pounds around the year-end holidays?

Some understanding of the digestive processes is a necessary part of knowing what happens to ingested food and in controlling one's weight. By presenting some of the basic knowns and suspicions, we hope to help in understanding, and perhaps help in moderating, the reader's approach to food. This kind of understanding can evolve into avoiding dietary recidivism, the biggest scourge of temporarily successful reducers.

Much of the information to be presented is fairly widely known to Physicians, Nurses, Physiologists, Dietitians, and many other Health Care professionals. Partial information is frequently found in the lay literature, unfortunately lacking completeness. The periodical press seems to be the source of much partially true information and a great deal of misinformation and misunderstanding which can lead to the lay reader's misguidance and frustration. If someone is burdened with excess weight, from a few to many extra pounds, even a partial understanding of nutritional and physiologic facts can help to provide a healthier weight! But the need for a complete and lasting revision of one's understanding of the nutrition process, including a permanent change in one's approach to food, becomes a major part of dealing with the burden of obesity.

Chapter 10

Physiology and Phases of Digestion, Basic Physiologic Concepts: Brief Overview of Phases of Eating and Digestion, Absorption & Utilization, Short and Long Term Storage

Cerebral and Oral Phases of Digestion

As a meal is contemplated, the digestive process actually begins. It probably starts with the sensation of hunger and triggers saliva and other digestive juice flows, very likely aided by good smells. When the physical ingestion of the food begins, the inborn act or reflex of swallowing is not the physical beginning of the process, but after placing the food in the mouth, the salivating and chewing is. Intact, or at least functioning, dentition naturally is an important part of this process. Cattle ranchers recognize this importance when they utilize false teeth to extend the lives of their cows. As the food is chewed, it is not only broken down into smaller, chemically accessible particles, but it becomes mixed with the first digestive secretions. The Saliva contains enzymes, mucous, and water secreted by the salivary glands, forming the food mixture into a semisolid bolus, which can then be swallowed. Our mothers' innate understanding of the importance of this process was frequently implied in repeated urgings to "chew your food!"

Gastric Phase

After arriving in the Stomach, the food bolus now becomes semi-liquid, while being churned and mixed with the stomach digestive juices, the stomach acid and mucus (or slime). The food, secretions, and water mixture is held temporarily in the stomach, and then is passed downwards in small amounts.

Small Intestinal Phase

After a varying period, depending on the size and content of the bolus, the food is passed on from the Stomach into the upper small intestine (Duodenum) in small amounts, where it is mixed with other juices produced by the most powerful digestive gland in the body, the Pancreas, and with Bile from the Liver. While the chemical environment in the Stomach is acidic, allowing the main gastric enzymes to function there most efficiently while the food is present, the pancreatic enzymes which chemically break down fats and further break down starches and proteins, in the Small Intestine work better in an alkaline environment. This is produced by the secretions first met in the Duodenum, both from the duodenal lining glands and from the Liver (Bile) and Pancreas (Pancreatic Juice).

Now partly mechanically, as well as chemically, broken down into their smaller molecular components, the nutrients in the duodenal bolus are forced downward into the Jejunum then into the Ileum by the peristaltic action of two layers of smooth or involuntary muscle lining the long hollow muscular gut tube. At the neither end of the Small Intestine, as the bolus progresses from the Ileum into the Large Intestine it is still semi-liquid. Although many of the now chemically separated nutrients have previously been absorbed via the approximately twenty feet of mucosal lining during passage through the Small Intestine. The swallowed water, water liberated from the food chemicals by digestive enzyme action, and the water contained in the various digestive juices remains mixed with the now nutrient depleted food and bacterial bolus (several species of bacteriae grow within the Intestine).

Interdigestive Phase

After the food and gastric secretions have mixed and then left the Stomach in small squirts the rest of the intestinal tract may still be processing the liquid bolus. During the day, although the Stomach may already be empty, the Small Intestine continues its peristaltic, secretory, and absorptive activity until the digestive process is completed. During the sleep period, the Small Intestine, then the entire body, gradually completes the digestive, absorptive, and storage phases. At this stage, sometimes designated "fasting," the individual is said to be in the "interdigestive phase."

Large Intestinal Phase

One result of the Darwinian selective process is seen when the bolus arrives in the Large Intestine. Following good conservation practices, most of the contained water in the food is now absorbed by the large intestinal lining, particularly on the right side of the Colon, creating the semisolid fecal mass with which we are all familiar. The final digestive phase is one of storage on the left side of the Large Intestine or Colon until a convenient time and place can be found for stool discharge, a process again involving a complex series of reflexes and voluntary actions, analogous to those of swallowing.

Absorption

As the several classes of food are being broken down into their smaller components by the various digestive processes and as the food and digestive juice mixture, or bolus, passes downward through the Stomach and Small Intestine, food absorption begins to take place through the gut mucosa. Although the process begins in the Stomach, most of it happens in the Small Intestine, the lining of which apparently varies in its ability to absorb various ingested materials.

Distribution

When the chemically broken down and now absorbed chemicals from the food enter the blood stream from the Stomach and Small Bowel, some of them are carried directly to the Liver by a special separate venous system, named for its main collecting vein, the Portal. Arriving in the Liver, the various chemicals are acted upon according to the body needs, certainly not by any volitional process. An important other pathway for the absorbed food chemicals is via the intestinal lymphatics, thence into the general circulation, bypassing the Liver on the first pass. If a peripheral requirement is sensed, the necessary chemical (be it one of the "essentials" or not) is usually distributed by dispatch from the Liver directly, into the blood stream and the general circulation via the regular Hepatic venous system. Entering the general circulation, the required substance eventually gets to wherever it is needed in the body.

Storage, Short Term

The Liver has been described as having "a thousand" functions. That estimate may be low. It certainly is the key participant in most metabolic processes relating to nutrition, serving and satisfying the several requirements without any conscious effort on the part of the owner. It is thought that the Liver also begins the storage function, if the body senses no immediate requirement for some of the atoms or molecules from the food which is being processed. For storage, it converts presently unneeded six carbon sugars (Chapter 2) into the multisugar starch, glycogen, and this starch is formed and stored temporarily in the Liver cells. When there is a peripheral requirement for sugar or immediate potential chemical energy, the Liver can also break down it's glycogen and provide sugar on demand to the general circulation. A very similar process is probably what happens to the other nutrients in our diet, both "essential" and non-essential. The particular "essential" components, be they molecular or atomic, are first presented to and temporarily stored in the Liver. Then, either via the Hepatic venous drainage or via the intestinal lymphatics (the second absorption route), thence into the general circulation, the required substance is delivered, ultimately to the needy cell. Exactly how or why the Liver responds to the various needs is mostly undetermined, but that this process is integral to food utilization is indisputable and the Liver digestive organ function is certainly indispensable.

Storage, Long Term

Excess nutrients or food potential energy not currently needed is stored in various sites until called for; how, nobody knows. If no immediate requirement exists for energy and energy excess to current needs is presented to the body through foods, the excess energy will be automatically stored in the most space-efficient or compact way available, namely in triglycerides in the fat (Chapter 4).

Although specific hormones and enzymes are apparently necessary for each of the various metabolic and storage processes to occur, as well as for the mobilization of required stores, if a requirement exists and if the stores are there, the normal body metabolism will mobilize them. But, if potential energy excess to the current need is taken in, it will be stored. Of course, when humans had a marginal or subsistence existence, this feature had real survival value. Plentiful food and the consequences attendant on increased energy storage are now being recognized as having a negative long term survival effect. As Dr. Atul Gewande so cleverly points out in his book, "Complications," "We are a species that has evolved to survive starvation, not to resist abundance." Picador Press 2003.

Chapter 11

Embryology, Endoderm, Mesoderm and Ectoderm, Development of the Pituitary Gland, Beyond Birth

The Beginning

In order to obtain some insight into and understanding of the body's workings, it is necessary to understand a little of how the body develops. Almost immediately after the egg is fertilized, the multipotential cells of the egg start to divide and rapidly grow. The first few cell divisions form a globe, which soon becomes hollow and the future embryo starts as a thickening or plate of cells on one side of the ball. This probably happens before the developing embryo becomes implanted in the lining of the mother's uterus.

The thickened layer of growing cells becomes two layers, called the outer or "ectoderm" and the inner or "endoderm". While continuing to grow, each of these layers begins to fold inward toward the other, finally forming a tube, the ectoderm eventually forming the skin, and the neural tube, from which the brain and spinal cord eventually develop. The endoderm forms the Gut and it's derivatives, including the Lungs and a part of the excretory system.

The cells growing between these two major layers, or "mesoderm," eventually form the skeleton, the muscles, the cardiovascular system (including the Heart), and other important body elements, including most of the fat storage cells. The sequence and other details of embryonic growth and development need not concern us here, but as the various tissues form and undergo very rapid growth, some resorption also normally occurs.

Also, some of the cells and tissues, particularly the nerve cells or their processes, migrate to new locations; in some cases they retain some of their original attachments. It is suspected that the blood forming cells start in the Placenta, move to the Liver in later fetal stages, then ultimately to the Bone Marrow. Other structures enlarge, then atrophy and are resorbed, and are normally completely gone by birth. If the normal resorption process is faulty, or if development stops at some point, serious congenital anomalies can and occasionally do occur.

Later Events: Endoderm, Mesoderm, Ectoderm

The inner Gut or endoderm lining forms the Stomach and intestinal lining or Mucosa, and endodermal branches form the Lungs and Liver. The middle embryonic cell layer, or mesoderm, contributes vessels and an inner circular and an outer longitudinal layer of "smooth" or involuntary muscle to the Gut. These smooth muscle tubes make up the bulk of the Gut, or gastrointestinal tract (called, for convenience, alimentary or GI tract). Blood vessels and lymph or tissue juice vessels develop just under the mucosal lining of the intestine to nourish the mucosal cells and to help drain absorbed digestive products. Some vessels eventually exit the forming body via the Umbilical Cord leading to and from the Placenta, where exchange of maternal nourishments, waste products, and Oxygen take place. Some blood vessels also form to enable the Fetal blood to nourish the gut muscles. Long ectodermal nerve cells, migrating, form their endings for sensation in the gut wall, growing between the smooth muscle fibers and deep to the mucosal lining. Other nerves (called the motor nerves) carry stimuli that cause the intestinal muscles to contract, but exactly why the coordination of contractions, called peristalsis, happens, causing the intestinal contents to be propelled downwards, is imperfectly understood.

Before development has proceeded very far, cavities form in the mesoderm around the Intestine, the Lungs and the forming Heart. The lining of the abdominal wall and the cavity surrounding the intestine becomes the Peritoneum. A fold of this lining, called the Omentum, containing fat cells, nerves, and blood vessels, drapes down over the front of the Large and Small Intestines from the Stomach. Because the peritoneal cover of the intestines is slippery and free, the contained viscera can move back and forth against each other as a peristaltic wave passes the food along within the Gut, although the intestine can do its digestive work, even if it is not entirely free.

The neural tube, by hugely growing in some areas while growing less rapidly or even resorbing in others forms the Brain and Spinal Cord (the beginnings of the central nervous system or CNS). Although incompletely formed at birth, recognizable adult features start to develop. Some of the nerve cells eventually are extremely long (up to a Meter). Non-nerve cells migrate (from the mesoderm) to form a support structure within and outside the Brain and Spinal Cord, containing arteries and veins as well as some of the ectoderm derived sensory nerves. Some of these cells provide various coverings of the CNS (called Meninges).

Some of the longer sensory nerves carry sensation directly back to the Brain from the limbs, usually with only one cell to cell link, as well as between the Intestine and the Brain. So-called "voluntary" motor nerves carry signals from the brain to "voluntary" or skeletal muscles, again with one or more links.

Autonomic Nervous System

"Involuntary" or "autonomic" nerves carry signals from deeper parts of the Brain to the "smooth" or involuntary muscles, particularly in the blood vessels, Lungs and Gut. Usually sensory nerve fibers from the Gut accompany the Autonomic Motor Nerves, and both frequently lie adjacent to blood vessels supplying the same part. The Autonomic Nerves also supply other organs, like the Heart and Lungs. As the Brain grows in the forming fetus, the highest centers for sensation, control, vision etc. form in the Cerebral Cortex. Just below the Cortex lies the next highest cerebral center, the Thalamus.

From animal studies, it is suspected that there are at least two thalamic centers which impact on eating. A center in the lateral Hypothalamus is apparently at least partially responsible for voracious eating, but stimulation of another center in the ventromedial Hypothalamus causes satiety-like behavior. Destruction of either center has the opposite effect (i.e. destruction of the lateral Hypothalamic center causes reduced food seeking behavior and destruction of the medial Hypothalamic center causes voracious eating). These centers also react to hormones brought to them by the blood and respond to some of the more modern diet moderating drugs, which apparently achieve their effects through these centers.

Development of the Pituitary Gland

Meanwhile, of course, the brain itself is growing and developing multiple connections, both to the rest of the body and to other parts of the brain. One of the better understood connections is to a tiny organ found at the base of the brain. This organ, the Pituitary Gland, has been thought to be the "master" hormone gland, apparently directing many of the other endocrine or "ductless" glands through its secretions, as well as elaborating growth hormone.

The posterior part of this organ is really a physical part of the Brain, with multiple connections to that part directly above it, the Thalamus. It is thought that the posterior or rear part of the Pituitary Gland, which is directly connected to the Thalamus by the Pituitary Stalk, directs hormone output from the Anterior Pituitary Gland in response to signals generated in the lower Thalamus. Then, via blood borne signals, messages are sent from the Posterior Pituitary to the Anterior Pituitary. Thus, a hunger or satiety signal may begin as a nerve impulse in the Thalamus and be converted to a hormonal signal by the Posterior Pituitary, thence be transmitted to the body by a different hormone arising from the Anterior Pituitary. Exactly how this process works has yet to be determined.

Beyond Birth

Obviously, after going through all the developmental changes before birth, the human baby, when born, still has a long growth and development phase ahead. For instance, three sets of Kidneys take part in the development of the Urogenital system prior to birth. Further growth and maturation still lie ahead after birth. Likewise, the brain is incompletely formed at birth and the growth, maturation, and the education process only begins before birth. It has been stated that the adult fat cells, or adipocytes, can multiply during the early years, but the number of these cells is fixed in the adult, yet, although fixed in number at an early age, they apparently can accommodate whatever storage demands are made on them.

Chapter 12

Oral Cavity: Saliva, Chewing, Swallowing, Esophagus, Lower Esophageal Sphincter, Vomiting

Oral Cavity

We are all familiar with the thought of "mouth watering" foods. This really is the result of mental stimulation of the flow of saliva, usually in response to thinking about, smelling or otherwise anticipating food. In effect, this saliva secretion is the true, physical beginning of the digestive process, before the first morsel of food is actually taken into the mouth.

Saliva

Saliva's composition varies, but it contains water, buffers to regulate pH or acidity, mucous, and the first digestive enzymes the food will meet in it's course through the intestinal tract.

Chewing

Two other important digestive functions occur in the mouth. Biting and chewing provide physical reduction of the larger pieces of food. Chewing, in concert with the cheeks and tongue causes mixing of the food and saliva secreted by the various Salivary Glands. This mechanical mixing exposes the food to the salivary digestive enzymes and starts the chemical breakdown process. Simultaneously, the mucous helps convert the solid food into a semi-solid and malleable, slippery mass that then can be readily swallowed.

The other important oral digestive function excites much speculation, but lacks firm factual footing. Most of the "taste buds" are found in the Tongue and taste has been shown to connect to the Brain via the Seventh (Facial), Ninth (Glossophryngeal), and Tenth (Vagus) Cranial Nerves. (The Eighth Cranial Nerve [Auditory] serves hearing and balance.) However, the taste buds in the Tongue have also been demonstrated to be limited in their appreciation of stimuli via the Twelfth (Hypoglossal) Nerve to sweet, bitter, salty, and sour. To fully appreciate flavor we apparently require an intact sense of smell which is transmitted via the First (Olfactory) Cranial Nerve. The degree of interdependence of these two senses has not been elucidated. How the central stimulation caused by taste or smell causes variation in Saliva composition also has not been determined, but that it does occur is well established.

Swallowing

When the food has been chewed and mixed with saliva, it is ready for the next step in the digestive process, swallowing. Although swallowing is a reflexive action that starts before birth, the initiation of swallowing can be voluntarily controlled. Innervated by the Twelfth Cranial Nerve, the Tongue is made up of several intertwining voluntary muscles, over which we have complete control. As food is chewed, the Tongue accommodates the bulk and, in concert with the cheeks, forces the mixture of food and saliva between the Molar Teeth to continue the grinding and mixing.

When the food bolus is ready to be swallowed, the Tongue senses the consistency of the air-food-saliva mixture and initiates the motile digestive process by forcing the semi-solid bolus back into the cavity behind the Tongue (Oropharynx). Several things happen, almost simultaneously, when this process begins.

The back part of the Tongue rises and creates a pressure which forces the food bolus into the posterior chamber behind the Tongue, the Oropharynx. The voluntary muscles in the soft Palate close off the chamber behind the nose

(Nasopharynx), preventing the food from rising up behind and into the nose. Almost at the same time, the cartilaginous trap door behind the Tongue (Epiglottis) falls over the upper opening of the voice box (Larynx), thereby preventing the food mixture from entering the windpipe (Trachea) and causing choking. At times, air is swallowed with the food or saliva, and this air is sometimes the greatest volume being swallowed. This can happen in the absence of food, but only with difficulty in the absence of saliva. Usually the food/saliva mixture enters the Esophagus without difficulty.

Esophagus

As the semi-solid food/saliva mixture is forced downwards into the upper part of the hollow muscular tube connecting the Mouth to the Stomach (the Esophagus or gullet), the smooth or involuntary muscles lining the tube take over. Henceforward the control of digestive passage of the nutrients becomes automatic, or Autonomic, as the controlling nerves leading to these smooth muscles are called.

Lower Esophageal Sphincter (LES)

At the lower end of the Esophagus, just beyond where the muscular tube passes through the Diaphragm, there is an anatomically poorly defined, yet very effective circular muscle, called the "Lower Esophageal Sphincter" or LES. This sphincter allows the semi-solid air-food-saliva mixture to pass into the Stomach by relaxing at just the right moment as the bolus approaches, and normally prevents Stomach contents from regurgitating, refluxing or rising back up into the Esophagus, Pharynx, or Mouth.

When we are about to vomit, the LES does seem to relax at exactly the right moment If one has a large amount of gas in the Stomach bubble, either by swallowing air or release of gas dissolved in a previously swallowed liquid, a similar reversal of the normal flow can take place. This is apparently under some sort of volitional abdominal wall muscle control, since this is the basis of suppression of socially unacceptable noise as well as Esophageal Speech, learned by some who have lost use of their voice boxes. Apparently a degree of increase in intraabdominal tension is involved in Esophageal speech, which can more readily be thought of as a controlled belch. But relaxation of the LES is an integral part of Esophageal Speech.

Vomiting

Vomiting is not a part of normal behavior. But when we are about to vomit, the LES does seem to relax at exactly the right moment. Whether caused by intra-gastric irritants, or by cerebral or other causes, the act of vomiting, although mostly involuntary, can be subject to some voluntary control. Signals for the non-voluntary part are probably sent through the Autonomic Nervous System. There is undoubtedly a considerable amount of coordination of signals required, since the LES must relax, the involuntary stomach wall muscles must contract, proba-bly the Pyloric (distal Stomach sphincter) also must contract, and the voluntary abdominal wall muscles controlling intraabdominal pressure must contract, all at just about the same time.

After passing through the LES, the food bolus enters the stomach.

Chapter 13

Stomach Anatomy, Gastric Digestion, Belching, Satiety, Delay of Emptying, Colic

Anatomy

An uninformed layperson thinks of the "Stomach" as that portion of the front of the body between the ribs and the pelvis. The anatomically informed refer to that area as the Anterior Abdominal Wall and know that the Abdominal Cavity lying just behind the Anterior Abdominal Wall contains most of the digestive organs, including the Stomach. The Skin, Subcutaneous Fat, Voluntary Muscles and their Fasciae, Parietal Peritoneum and other structures make up the abdominal wall envelope which encloses and contains most of the digestive organs and others (like the Omentum, Kidneys, Spleen, Bladder and Uterus).

An increase in the thickness of the subcutaneous fat in the Abdominal Wall and increased fat deposition in the peritoneal apron (Omentum) suspended below the Stomach, but within the Peritoneal Cavity and in front of and below the Transverse Colon become a significant part of the "large stomach" or "big belly" associated with obesity.

Gastric Digestion

After being chewed, mixed with saliva, and swallowed, food proceeds into the Stomach (Latin: Gaster), past the LES into the next, wider part of the hollow Gut tube below the Esophagus. Here, the digestive process begins in earnest. Although the Stomach size can be quite variable (normally it can readily hold a couple of quarts). It can also become much more commodious and does in some disease states. The Stomach lining (Gastric Mucosa) secretes several substances which mix with the contained food to break down the food chemicals into smaller, more readily absorbable forms. Among the Gastric secretions are water, hydrochloric acid and digestive enzymes which begin to break down chemically the ingested starches and proteins into some of their components.

Mixing and churning of the Stomach contents is helped by the contraction of interlocking involuntary smooth muscle fibers in the wall of the Stomach itself, which are under Autonomic Nervous System control. This is the real beginning of peristalsis or coordinated active food propulsion downwards. The rate and type of mucosal secretions and the intrinsic muscular action are under the control of various circulating hormones and the Autonomic Nervous System with the contents-sensing mechanism of the Stomach as the first part of the automatic or Autonomic Sensory Nerve-Brain-Autonomic Motor Nerve loop.

Absorption of the chemically broken down food molecules begins in the Stomach. While in the Stomach, the food becomes further mixed with the digestive secretions, and becomes more liquid in the process. The churning taking place here allows better contact between the Gastric digestive enzymes which function best in the acidic (low pH) and liquefied environment within that organ and the partially broken down potential energy bearing chemicals in the food.

Belching

"Gas" occurring in the Stomach is not usually the result of fermentation, but primarily swallowed air. Although the sensation of swallowing saliva, ice chips or water leads one to think that very little air is going into the Stomach, actually, the reverse is true. On the other hand, Carbon Dioxide (CO_2) gas dissolved in cold soda, which has been warmed in the Stomach then released from solution is actually in liquid form when swallowed. When the Stomach bubble above the liquid contents becomes larger than the wall can comfortably accommodate, the air or warmed Carbon Dioxide is released and it rises into the throat, usually accompanied by a noise. Gastric gas, not escaping upwards, is mixed with the gastric contents and discharged downwards into the small intestine.

Occasionally, we become aware of muscle contractions in the Stomach wall, and we quickly come to associate that sensation from the Stomach Wall muscle contraction with an empty organ, perhaps even before birth. As these intrinsic stomach muscles contract we sense the churning and, whether the Stomach needs to be filled or not, we assume it does. This is the first physiologic foundation of my thesis, found in the book's title. If there is much air in the Stomach when this happens, we will hear "growling," or gas churning, almost continuously, although some of that noise may be arising from the more distal parts of the Small or Large Intestine.

Satiety

Another sensation, apparently arising from the Stomach, is one of satiety or "fullness". Whether this comes solely from the sensors within the Stomach wall, from hormonal response to digestive products in the blood stream (thence to the Brain), to a combination of these factors, or to some other influence or combination is not known.

It is fairly well established that the capacity of a fasting Stomach will decline quite quickly or "shrink" within a few days of the fast's beginning, and the sensation of Hunger will be felt no longer. On the other hand, the presence of either proteins or fats in the partially digested food within the Stomach or in the Small Intestine immediately below slows the rate of Gastric wall muscle contraction and has the effect of retarding the emptying of the Stomach. This may be a source of the sense of satiety. However, a sense of satiety does not arise from an empty stomach.

Delay of Emptying

Inhibition of Stomach motility caused by the presence of protein or fat within the Stomach contents or Duodenum, probably explains why most Chinese food, known to be relatively low in fat and protein and high in carbohydrates, may lead to the widely held belief that Chinese food doesn't stay with you very long. Unfortunately, delay of Stomach emptying also provides ample maneuvering room for charlatans, touting the advantages of a high protein or high fat diet to delay Gastric emptying and associated hunger sensations, while ignoring their expense and the high caloric content, particularly in high fat diets, along with the other established downsides of high fat consumption.

That thought processes influence the Stomach is readily understood. We have only to recall that when one is hungry, merely thinking about food can cause appreciable and sensed Stomach muscle activity. This activity is probably under the influence of the Tenth Cranial Nerve (Vagus, part of the Brain and Autonomic Nervous System) leading directly to and from the Brain to the Stomach and other organs. (For further discussion of Brain effects, see Chapter 16.) This can also occur involuntarily, i.e. without thinking about food.

Colic

Most hollow organs have sensory elements in their walls which can only tell us that the wall is being stretched. When a hollow viscus is stretched intermittently, as by the passage of a normal peristaltic wave along the wall, a local buildup of pressure is normal and without symptoms. When partial blockage occurs, the abnormally higher intraluminal pressure stretches the wall muscle and compresses the sensory nerve endings. This is interpreted as pain, and a series of these pains is called "cramps" or "colic". Described as one of the worst pains known to man, acute blockage of the hollow tube leading from the Kidney down to the Urinary Bladder (Ureter), as by a stone, causes a similar pain, called in this case, Renal (Kidney) Colic.

Complete Stomach blockage rarely occurs, but blockage farther down the hollow intestinal tract does occur occasionally and can cause similarly severe cramps, in this case called "Intestinal Colic". The first response to partial hollow organ blockage is smooth muscle contraction in the organ wall. By failing to overcome a chronic partial blockage, the smooth muscle in the wall above the obstruction works harder to increase the intraluminal pressure, and in the attempt to overcome a chronic obstruction the wall muscle hypertrophies. If a portion of the Gut tube is not working (aperistaltic), a functional obstruction exists. This is thought to be the cause of cramping or "Intestinal Colic" experienced with acute food poisoning or post-operative cramping. When several scattered portions of the Intestine are paralyzed simultaneously while other parts above the non-working parts of the tube are contracting, "Colic" can occur. Chronic failure to eliminate an obstruction, with its accompanying wall stretching is thought to be the source of a repeated cramping sensation. In long standing chronic partial hollow organ obstruction, the proximal smooth muscle wall usually hypertrophies. Intestinal Colic resulting from partial small bowel obstruction can, in turn, set up stomach muscle contractions, probably reflexly through the Autonomic Nervous System.

The Gastric or intestinal contractions can even be sent backwards; a condition known as reverse peristalsis. This may result in vomiting, even what has been described as "fecal vomiting." although that may be a misnomer. Of course, vomiting is not a normal process, but it usually requires combined voluntary and involuntary as well as cerebral coordination.

Although much has been learned over time about how the Stomach and Intestine function together, I doubt that any knowledgeable person would be willing to state that there is no more to be learned. Medicine has been called an inexact science and most experienced practitioners will agree with that. On the other hand, the material which has already been learned allows us to make some of what are probably a first approximations to the truth. That yet to be learned factors exist will not be denied, but "unknown" is not equal to "unknowable". Unproven conjecture on the other hand, may be and frequently is the starting point for new information. However, one must guard against drawing unsubstantiated conclusions based on unproven conjectures.

Next

Having been processed in the Stomach and prepared for further chemical breakdown and absorption of nutrients, the food now leaves the Stomach little by little and enters the Duodenum through the Stomach's distal circular muscle called the Pylorus.

Chapter 14

Small Intestinal Factors: Duodenum, Jejunum, Ileum, Absorption, Bile in Fat Digestion and Enterohepatic Recirculation of Bile Salts, Autonomic Innervation, Intrinsic Hormones, Colon, Rectum and Anus

Duodenum

Entering the next part of the intestinal tract below the Stomach, the now partially digested, liquefied and acidified food mixture is metered into the Duodenum in frequent small amounts through a thickening of the circular Stomach muscle exit called the Pylorus. Exactly how the Pylorus functions is not completely understood, but the Pylorus does seem to relax and allow repeated passage of small food amounts from the Stomach into the Duodenum.

After secretion by the Liver, alkaline Bile is stored and concentrated in the Gall Bladder between meals. This concentrated Bile is squirted into the Duodenum and mixed with the food, as it first arrives in the Duodenum. The very strong alkaline digestive juice secreted by the Pancreas also enters the Duodenum, usually via the same tubular opening in the Duodenal wall through which the Bile enters. The Bile concentrating Gall Bladder function apparently is not essential to digestion, since Gall Bladder removal is well tolerated, and normal digestion can proceed without that first blast of concentrated Gall Bladder Bile. As more and more of the mixed food and Gastric Juice enters through the Pylorus, more dilute Bile continues to be secreted by the Liver during the digestive process. This more dilute Bile flows directly from the Liver into the Duodenum via the Common Bile Duct.

The enzymes, or digestant factors in the Pancreatic and small intestinal lining secretions require an alkaline environment to function best in breaking down the various food molecules. Bile helps provide this environment. The process continues until the Stomach is empty.

Jejunum and Ileum

Meanwhile, the intestinal lining (Mucosa) is beginning to absorb some of the now chemically broken down, smaller food molecules and atoms. The folds of the inner intestine lining resemble wet velvet in appearance and feel. The Small Intestinal Mucosal surface area which does the nutrient absorption is said to be several times greater than the area of skin (1.7 square Meters Skin Area in the average 70Kg man). As the food-digestive juice-gas combination passes downward in the Small Intestine through the Jejunum and then the Ileum, increasing amounts of the ingested foods are broken down chemically into their components, and then absorbed.

Absorption

Apparently, different substances are taken up through the Mucosa at different levels of the Small Intestine, although this is a mostly unknown subject. Unfortunately, it was discovered some time ago that so-called "intestinal short-circuiting," or bypassing for morbid or intractable obesity had deleterious and unanticipated bad effects, particularly when certain segments of the Small Intestine were bypassed. Therefore, this procedure has fallen into appropriate disrepute for serious weight control sufferers.

Starches and Proteins are soluble in the enteric water environment and thus are accessible to their particular digestive enzymes (Amylases and Peptidases, respectively) for chemical dissection, or breakdown, in preparation for absorption. After this preparation, the smaller, water soluble food components are transported across the Mucosal Cell lining and thence into the Portal Blood or Lymphatics and eventually to the Liver.

Bile in Fat Digestion and Enterohepatic Recirculation of Bile Salts

Because they are not soluble in water, fats require different handling to be entered into the body's internal environment (strictly speaking, the Gut lumen is external to the body's internal environment). Lipids undergo emulsification in preparation for absorption. Specific, so-called "Bile Salts", secreted by the Liver (Taurocholic and Glycocholic Acid Salts), allow food fat molecules (Triglycerides, Cholesterol and its esters, Phospholipids; see Chapter 4) to be suspended in the aqueous environment of the Small Intestine and then allow the larger molecules to be attacked by lipase enzymes. The Bile Salts also allow for the transport and then delivery of fat molecules across the Mucosal cells. In this process the Bile salts are returned to the Liver, where they are separated from the digested food fat by the Liver cells and re-excreted in the Bile. This travel is referred to as the Enterohepatic circulation of Bile Salts.

Some of the Vitamins (A, D, E, & K) are fat-like in their solubility. Their absorption into the body's internal milieu is dependent on the functional adequacy of the enterohepatic fat absorption mechanism. The part bacteriae play in vitamin production within the intestine is suspected, but unknown.

Autonomic Innervation

There are two sets of "Automatic" or Autonomic Motor nerves which supply the intestinal tract. Some of the motor fibers cause muscle contractions and peristalsis, others digestant fluid secretions. Both motor autonomic systems are accompanied by sensory fibers that carry back information, usually along the same peripheral nerve pathways as the motor nerves, and eventually back to the Brain. It is thought that these nerves are only capable of reporting a buildup of pressure within the hollow organ they innervate, but this is not an established fact.

Intrinsic Hormones

In addition to neuroactive communications secretions (Chapters 10, 16), three other kinds of cell secretions are recognized, two for communication, one for work:

Exocrine: Cell Secretions which are carried to another area remote from the source cell, usually via hollow tubes of cells or "Ducts". Groups of exocrine secreting cells are called Exocrine Glands (e.g. Various digestive glands). Similarly, other exocrine glands perform other functions like sweat and milk formation.

Endocrine: Chemical molecules which act as signals are usually secreted from one special gland cell and sent to another target cell, usually remote, via the circulating blood. (These constitute the so-called "Ductless Glands".) Groups of specific hormone secreting cells are usually named by their source locations (e.g. Pituitary, Thyroid or Adrenal Cortex).

Paracrine: Endocrine signals usually elaborated and targeted on an adjacent cell (e.g. Intestinal Mucosa gland secretions).

In addition, "Autocrine" mechanisms are described, but at least a semantic case can be made against a special cell function which acts within itself, since in any multicellular organism each cell may have more than one type of function. At one time endocrine secretions were all considered to be under the control of the Pituitary Gland, but some of the gastrointestinal hormones, like Gastrin and Cholecystokinin (CCK) are elaborated in the Duodenal Wall without apparent Pituitary influence. Resultant actions, like acid production from the Stomach Mucosal glands or Gall Bladder wall muscle contraction, respectively, follow blood borne transport of each signal. Thus, these signals fit the endocrine definition, but apparently are beyond Pituitary control.

Large Intestine (Colon)

Having passed through the Small Intestine, been chemically split into smaller molecules and subjected to absorption, the now nutritionally depleted intestinal contents enter the Large Intestine or Colon. In the right side of the Large Intestine, the water contained in the food and digestive juice is conserved by being absorbed, thereby converting the bowel contents into a semi-solid mass.

Some of the Large Intestinal Mucosa cells secrete mucus which has the effect of lubricating the stool.

The left side of the Large Intestine is thought to play a primary storage role; holding digestive residue until it can be conveniently disposed of. At this point, the food chemicals minerals and water have not only been almost totally absorbed, but the bulk of the Large Intestinal contents here are (about 95%) various bacteriae.

Fiber, another word for plant celluloses, is humanly indigestible, but adds to the bulk of the stool by attracting water. This happens both by intrinsic volume increase from the fiber and by increasing the water content. Increasing stool bulk primarily by fiber ingestion is thought to confer some health benefits, again strongly suspected, but not proven.

The functions of bacteria within the GI tract are not well understood, but the presence of several varieties of bacteriae within the human gut lumen at least requires various surgical adaptations, particularly when dealing with the Colon. Interestingly, the human portal vein blood and liver are sterile. In dogs, on the other hand, they are not. Why? Who knows.

Rectum and Anus

Stool passage occurs as another combination of voluntary and involuntary behavior (comparable to swallowing). In the Anus another distinct circular muscle is found; this one described as being the only muscle in the body capable of distinguishing water from air. Feces can also be a major route for the body to rid itself of unwanted toxic substances. These are usually placed in the intestine by the Liver via the Bile after detoxification and not later absorbed. Discharging undigested (e.g. fiber) or unabsorbed foods and swallowed air or gas formed during digestion and forced downwards in the intestinal tract by peristalsis, is also accomplished after storage in the Descending Colon, to be discharged at a socially convenient time. Although burdened with usually odiferous fermentation products (like Hydrogen Sulfide), the Colonic gas discharged by this route is largely swallowed air.

Chapter 15

Liver and Pancreas: Absorption, Liver Starch, Liver Metabolism, Detoxification and Excretion, Pancreas, Islets

Absorption

Other very significant factors enter into the digestive process. Chemically dissected or "digested" foods pass through the Intestinal wall by the active (or energy using) process called "absorption". The simpler smaller food molecules (Sugars, Amino Acids and Fatty Acids) and the single mineral atoms actually enter the body's own internal environment itself either via the blood veins or the tissue juice channels called "Lymphatics", within the intestinal wall just below the lining mucosa. Before this happens, although the various nutrients are within the intestinal lumen, they and the bacteria with them are truly outside the body's internal environment itself, and thus, not actually an integral part of the body.

The blood and lymphatic fluid draining the intestine, now rich in chemically broken down or digested and then absorbed food, drains either directly into the Liver via the separate venous system called the Portal, or through the lymphatic channels which flow upwards through the chest to empty into the blood stream above the Heart.

Liver

Although classification of Liver functions is susceptible to oversimplification, there are two primary ones, digestion and excretion. The Liver, the first organ the nutrient containing blood meets after leaving the digestive tract, has been suspected of and called many things. Here, storage of currently excess or unneeded energy or food molecules begins. When demanded elsewhere, the food or energy containing molecules are distributed to all parts of the body via the systemic blood vessels, starting with the Hepatic Veins. Then each cell in the body takes whatever it currently needs when the needed substance passes by in the nearby blood. If there are no current requirements, the Liver saves and converts excess food energy by manufacturing and storing sugars in the form of liver starch, or glycogen, a very complex carbohydrate.

Starch

The Liver starch can readily be converted back by the Liver cells into it's component sugars if required, either for immediate energy use or for structural purposes. The Liver cells also seem to be able to manufacture most of the non-essential amino acids and cholesterol, and will provide needed protein parts from the amino acids, if available. By definition, the Liver cannot manufacture the "essential" amino acids, although if it contains previously digested essentials, it can provide them for the needed peptides or proteins to be made up from the amino acids, either in the Liver or elsewhere until the amino acid supply is exhausted. Obviously, the other essentials, minerals for example, cannot be provided without an adequate supply in storage or in the current intake.

The manufacture and use of glycogen is a hugely complex subject, but it requires the presence of the hormone Insulin. Diabetics, lacking adequate amounts of this hormone, tend to have poor liver glycogen use, but consideration of that disease is well beyond our compass. Just as clearly, other effects of that too common disease impact on nutrition, not always in well understood ways.

Liver Metabolism

In the digestive process, the food chemicals (Starches, Proteins, and Fats), now broken down into their simplest component forms (Sugars, Amino Acids, and Fatty Acids) and the other "essentials," after being absorbed are either temporarily stored in the Liver or used at once. Liver Starch (Glycogen) is manufactured here, and some energy is consumed to perform this manufacture. Since there are no unique food ingredients required to perform this task for Carbohydrates, the Liver cells don't have to wait for the right ingredients to come along, but can proceed as the need presents. Some of the intricate chemical steps of Glycogen production have been worked out. In the Liver, the steps seem to be reversible, since the Liver can convert its Glycogen back to Sugar in response to the body's demand, other factors being equal (i.e. no diabetes). Incidentally, this raises the question of the veracity of that overworked diagnosis Low Blood Sugar, or "Hypoglycemia", since normal conversion of Liver glycogen to glucose should avoid too low a blood sugar.

Muscle cells can also form and store glycogen, although they cannot reconvert it back into sugar or mobilize it back into the blood, as can the Liver cells. Muscle glycogen is used for the work of energy production, when the muscle cells are called on to function.

In protein and fat utilization, the Liver's role is less well defined, but undoubtedly of similar importance. However, with these classes of chemicals, the requirements of the entire body must be met, and there may be a specific internal requirement of the Liver as well. Certainly starvation or non-starvation deprivation (for instance of certain nutrients) can cause disease development, either in the Liver or elsewhere.

Detoxification and Excretion

The main excretory product of the Liver, the Bile, normally contains various chemicals which act like detergents, aiding the fat digesting enzymes in the Pancreatic and intestinal juices in their enzymatic digestive assault on the fatty chemicals in the food.

Liver cells can also capture, detoxify, and excrete various poisons, although this is not a primary nutritional function. Thus, Liver detoxification may be thought of as an excretory function. However, if the toxin is poisonous to the Liver cells, they are more likely to be damaged because of their position as the first cells in line after toxin absorption. The Bile Salts, after aiding in the absorption of separated fat molecules, are removed from complexes in the blood by the Liver, then re-excreted in the bile (see Enterohepatic recirculation. in Chapter 14).

Pancreas

Anatomically speaking, the Pancreas is really two glands in one. The external or exocrine secretions contain the strongest digestive juices the body produces, capable of breaking down all three of the major chemical classes of food. Each digestive Pancreatic enzyme (amylase, protease, and lipase) breaks down one of the major food components (carbohydrates, proteins, and fats, respectively) within the upper Small Intestine, preparing the food chemicals for the next digestive phase, absorption. Most of the Pancreatic Gland substance is made up of this exocrine or externally secreting tissue which responds to both neurogenic and hormonal (or blood borne) instructions. The digestive fluids produced are conducted into the intestinal lumen by a series of internal tubes or "ducts".

Pancreatic Islets

Not connected to the intestine by ducts, but scattered throughout the gland, although concentrated in the tail of the organ, are little "islands" or nests of three types of cells that produce hormones. The Pancreatic Islets produce the hormones Insulin (from what are called Beta cells), Glucagon (from the Alpha cells), and Somatostatin (from the Delta cells). These hormones enter the blood directly and affect every cell in the body.

The two former hormones directly affect the way the body cells handle the sugar in the blood, and undoubtedly have other major influences on health, particularly Insulin, or more specifically, its lack. Although detailed consideration of Pancreatic function and malfunction is well beyond our subject, the gland's importance in the general digestive scheme is a significant, albeit dispensable one, and an important part of any discussion of digestion. Consequently, an understanding of its contribution is vital.

Chapter 16

Other Structures and Their Functions: Intercellular Communication and Cell Signals; CNS: Brain and Spinal Cord in Signal Interpretation, Brain Sensing; Sub-cortical Brain, Pituitary Gland and Hormones; Autonomic Nervous System, GI Reflexes, Thirst, Hunger, Satiety, Brain Information Handling, Fear, Theories

Cell Signals and Intercellular Communication

In any multicellular organism communication between cells is necessary for survival; the higher the complexity of the organism, the more pressing the need. Man, the most complex animal, has evolved two main methods of transmitting information between cells. Both the Circulatory and Nervous Systems spread chemical signals throughout the entire body. The Nervous System provides the most rapid and direct connections. Nerve cells, some almost a meter long, carry signals within themselves, then elaborate special chemicals at their endings to carry ongoing signals across tiny (10-100 nanometer) gaps between them and their target cells, be they other nerve cells, muscle cells, gland cells, or others. The Endocrine System sends other special secretions, called "Hormones," to various remote cells via the Blood. Some of the signals stimulate action in the target cells, others inhibit their function, whatever it is. Each of the endocrine cells generates a different chemical signal (hormone), called a "transmitter," recognizable by the specialized target cell. The nerves stimulate the various specialized tissue cells, as do several hormones, by lodging signals at specific receptor sites on the target cells. Some of the signals cause a "turn on" of the target cell effect, while others cause a "turn off" or down regulation of the effect. Among the neurotransmitters are the substances called Acetylcholine, Dopamine, Serotonin, and Noradrenalin. There are many hormones and some of the neurotransmitters are also thought to function as hormones. The target cells can be other nerve cells, for instance, in the Brain, and cells anywhere in the GI tract, mouth to anus, or elsewhere.

Although sending messages via nerves is the most rapid means of communication, hormonal chemical signals, carried to almost all parts of the body by the blood, are somewhat less rapid than the nerve signals, but just as effective.

Adult Brain and Spinal Cord (CNS Central Nervous System)

Previously (see Chapter 11) we have briefly described the development of the Brain and Spinal Cord. In the long and incompletely understood history of human species development, the crowning achievement probably has been our species evolution of its nervous system, particularly the Brain. Although many of the intimate functions of the intracerebral connections, suspected on the basis of demonstrated anatomic connections, remain to be worked out, there can be little doubt that the cerebral tissue is the ultimate controller of most of our various thoughts and actions. Regarding performance of it's role of highest controller within each body, a vital part must be the gathering of information from the body's furthest reaches, processing that information consciously or unconsciously, and then generating appropriate action on the basis of the information received and processed. Where or how the higher cerebral centers influence our behavior is the subject of intense speculation and some study. That Brain function controls behavior is not disputed.

Brain Sensing of Needs

Exactly where in the body the need for some food is sensed is really not known, but that the Brain is the final pathway for the sensing of several needs, among them the need for food, seems indisputable. Whether the Brain senses a need for sugar in the blood, food in the Stomach, water, warmth, sleep, or some other requirement is moot. Clearly, some of these requirements are manifested directly through sensory nerve connections, primarily via the autonomic pathways. Just as clearly, there are both sugar and hormones like Insulin and Glucagon circulating, which indicate that a requirement exists. In addition to reflex and hormonal sensing, there may also be an intrinsic direct Brain effect (psychological). Hormones signaling hunger apparently are elaborated in the Brain and elsewhere and targeted there also.

Sub-cortical Brain

Just below the highest Cerebral Brain Cortex, and intimately connected to it, lies the highest part of the brain stem, the Thalamus. Because the human brain is difficult to study, animal studies are used. From them, it is suspected that there are at least two thalamic centers that impact on eating. A center in the lateral Hypothalamus is apparently at least partially responsible for voracious eating, but stimulation of another center in the ventromedial Hypothalamus causes satiety-like behavior. Destruction of either center has the opposite effect, or destruction of the lateral Hypothalamic center causes reduced food seeking behavior and destruction of the medial Hypothalamic center causes voracious eating. These centers also react to hormones brought to them by the blood and they respond to some of the more modern diet moderating drugs that achieve their effects through these centers. Just below the Thalamus is the Pituitary Gland. The posterior part of this gland is really an extension of the Brain, with multiple connections to the Thalamus directly above. It is thought that the posterior or rear part of the Pituitary gland, directly connected to the Thalamus by the nerves in the Pituitary Stalk, directs output from the Anterior Pituitary Gland via blood borne chemical signals sent from the posterior part of the gland to the Anterior Pituitary, where Anterior Pituitary hormones are generated to be circulated throughout the body and, particularly, to the other endocrine glands. Also, a hunger or satiety signal might begin as a nerve impulse in the Thalamus and be converted to a hormonal signal in the Posterior Pituitary, then sent to the Anterior Pituitary and then returned to the Brain via another blood-borne signal.

Brain and Spinal Cord in Signal Interpretation

The Brain is the ultimate recipient of sensations arising in the Gastrointestinal Tract, usually carried back via the Spinal Cord or by the Vagus (Tenth Cranial) Nerve. The Brain is also the prime source of much of the activity stimulated following the GI input, although we may not be aware of it as it happens. Voluntary muscles at both ends of the GI tract are stimulated by a different type of nerve signal arising in the Brain. Less directly responsive, the involuntary muscles of most of the GI tract are subject to impulses carried through the Autonomic Nerve System.

Autonomic Nerve System

There are two sets of motor automatic or Autonomic Nerve Systems supplying most of the intestinal tract. Each motor system is called either "adrenergic" or "cholinergic," depending on their anatomic pathways and on the different chemical signals elaborated at their target ends. "Involuntary" or "autonomic" nerves carry signals from deeper parts of the brain to the "smooth" or involuntary muscles scattered throughout the body, particularly in the blood vessels, Lung and Gut. Both sets of efferent involuntary motor nerves are accompanied by sensory fibers. These sensory (afferent) Autonomic fibers carry information back mostly along the same peripheral nerve pathways as the motor (efferent) fibers, ultimately to the Brain. In response, some motor fibers cause involuntary gut muscle contractions, others various digestant fluid secretions. It is thought that the afferent Autonomic Sensory Nerves are only capable of reporting a buildup of pressure within each hollow organ innervated, but this is not an established fact. We do know that sensations arising from the hollow organs are transmitted through the Autonomic sensory fibers before a response is initiated.

GI Reflexes

Since the existence of Autonomic Sensory paths is well established, some of the responses are considered likely true. A good example of this is the response called "The Gastro-Colic Reflex." In this reflex, a full, or partially full Stomach is thought to trigger a sudden urge to evacuate the Colon. Another example occurs when a chronic partial blockage of the intestine stimulates enlargement of the involuntary gut wall muscles upstream from the blockage. This happens apparently without any awareness of the process on the part of the affected individual.

Thirst

It seems to be true that there are two main sensations for alimentation persisting into adulthood. Thirst is a very strong, almost undeniable, feeling that is usually associated with the body's perceived need for water. Although we come to associate the sensation with a dry mouth, we actually sense the need for water in our brains. Children, at a very early age, learn that asking for water tends to be a request which is universally accepted and which will be quickly satisfied, particularly at night. That the request may also become a manipulative opportunity is soon recognized both by the caregiver and the child. Yet, both the caregiver and child recognize the validity of the need in some way, although the responses of either may vary.

Hunger

A very basic need we all feel is a sense of hunger. What constitutes "hunger" or what it is, is not known. Next to thirst, it is probably the most urgent feeling many of us will ever experience, although there certainly are others. We do know that sensations can arise from the hollow organs, but exactly what constitutes "hunger" is not known. Specifically, what it is that makes us think we are hungry is not known, although it is probably a combination of knowing when our last meal was, what it was, how much of it there was, and how satisfied we were after eating it. Add to this our belief that in order to stay healthy we need to eat every few hours while we are awake and the uncomfortable sensation arising when we "owe" the stomach some food leads us to say we are hungry. The level of Gastric acidity may also have a role in sensing hunger and there probably are other contributing factors. If we hear "growling," or become aware of gas being moved about within the Gut, we are more readily persuaded that we need to eat. Although actual pain can arise from the stomach, frequently the discrimination between pain and hunger is not done. To avoid overeating, it is necessary to distinguish between pain and hunger. The saying that "hunger makes the best sauce" implies that a good appetite will overcome most idiosyncratic and imagined food preferences and will cause a truly hungry person to eat. Unfortunately, neither the recency nor the quantity or type of food consumed give reliable indications of when we should eat again and how much or what we should plan on taking in.

Satiety

The word "satiety" is derived from the Latin language and implies fullness to a satisfactory level. The word "surfeit" implies fullness to the point of overindulgence. Both words are used almost interchangeably, but the latter is more pejorative. In a previous paragraph in this chapter we mentioned the various sources of sensations that are sent to and perceived in various parts of the Brain. Is satiety a learned behavior? Does it really have anything to do with a full (i.e. stretched) Stomach wall? The Surgeons who form a much smaller food reservoir (+/-golf ball size) in the Stomachs of their morbidly obese patients by various means claim that the "full feeling" experienced by their patients cause them to voluntarily limit their food intake. The actual case may be that the consequences of stretching that small reservoir (nausea, regurgitation, and discomfort, if not actual pain) are less bearable than the satisfaction to be derived from further eating. Whatever the reason, we know that this approach has met with success. We don't yet know what the long term consequences or downsides of the various operations are.

Brain Information Handling and Psychological Considerations

Prominent among the many mental factors which can impact on the development or persistence of obesity are:

Frustration: Unbiased information is difficult to find. This book is an attempt to gather available facts in a useful form, particularly for those desiring basic nutritional understanding.

Embarrassment: In spite of recognizing the presence of a problem, the overweight and obese are usually reluctant to admit the problem to anyone other than their Physician.

Lack of Knowledge: The long-term dangerous consequences of obesity are increasingly publicized, but frequently denied by those most seriously afflicted.

Presence of a "Facilitator": Historical searching usually reveals someone in the immediate background or environs of the overeater. This facilitator supports an overeating and/or under exercising habit, or both.

Fear

Fears exist and they can be overwhelming in trying to correct inappropriate alimentation, such as:

"If I don't eat, I'm afraid something bad will happen."

"If I don't eat, I might die."

"I need to eat."

"I get dizzy when I don't eat."

"I don't feel good when I don't eat."

"I do feel good when I do eat."

Although reasonable, these statements are the product of a lack of understanding of the facts presented here and resistance of the overeater to change.

Theories

Various theories exist that attempt to explain the overeating/underutilizing behavior of obesity. Among them are an Overeating Compulsion, usually found in persons who, while being brought up, have been taught to "Clean off your plate!" complying with that ingrained directive. Also, there is the "Reinforcement Theory," which holds that certain additives or flavor enhancers provide immediate gratification of the eating urge. Some of these theories may also be operating in the very young child who associates comfort, warmth, and pleasant noises with a full stomach. Other theories exist which may prove to be true.

Chapter 17

Definitions and Psychology: Health, Obesity, Criticism, Hunger, Beginnings of Hunger Learning, Manipulative and Social Aspects of Food, Pressures to Eat, Conditioned Responses to Food, Excess Energy Storage, Obsessions and Compulsions, Anxieties, Binges, Denial, Water Confusion and Denial, Dietary Recidivism

Health

Except by exclusion, we lack a good definition for "Good Health". Although described as the absence of disease, everyone seems to understand what a state of "good health" is. The accompanying feeling of satisfaction, both physical and mental, seems also to be widely accepted as an integral part of "good health". There seems to be a part of our Brain that recognizes the "good" feeling, and there is animal evidence that this may occur in the Hypothalamus (see Chapter 16). Because substances capable of stimulating these areas have been shown to collect there, it has been postulated that an eventual role for medication can be discovered which will use this information. The neurotransmitter substance called "Serotonin" has been implicated in this response, and one of the sites of its action is thought to be the medial part of the Hypothalamus.

Obesity

Like the lack of a firm definition for "Good Health," we have no universally accepted definition for "Obesity," although both terms are generally understood. In the past, Life Insurance Tables have provided some guidelines, but the most readily available measure, the Body Mass Index [Wt (Kg)/Ht (M) x Ht (M)], although easy to compute, does not come with any standard. This situation is not all bad, since each adult must decide for him or herself what his or her weight should be. However, going to a predetermined target weight bracket and staying there has been and continues to be a difficult, frustrating, and trying, if not emotionally draining and harrowing experience. Our hope is that by developing an understanding of some of the chemistry and physiology involved a lay-person struggling with a weighty burden may be able to overcome the problem.

Since there is no universally accepted method for deciding at what level one's weight should be, just as there is none for achieving control of one's weight, each adult has to make this decision for him-or her-self. In arriving at a decision, it can be most helpful for an individual to understand that he or she has ultimate control of this decision. The need to accept the responsibility for that decision and the accompanying need to persevere for life can be most difficult and unpleasant to contemplate. As well, the potential rewards like improved self-image, lower chance of severe diabetes, lower blood pressure, and lower risk of coronary or other artery disease and untimely death, among others, and the lack of any immediate reward can be difficult to appreciate.

Criticism

It is easy to criticize people who are heavy, particularly if the critic is not, and most particularly if the critic has a history of obesity. One might expect greater understanding and tolerance from successful reducers, but successful reducers seem to have their favorite method which worked for them and which they vociferously advocate. Recipients of this criticism may seem to be very insensitive, but may well be adopting an appearance of indifference as a defense.

Hunger

The Oxford English Dictionary defines hunger as "the uneasy or painful sensation caused by want of food," and The American Heritage College Dictionary, 2nd Edition, says hunger is "a strong desire for food" or "the discomfort, weakness or pain caused by a lack of food". The parts of the definitions referring to an absence of recent food intake, and the accompanying "discomfort" or "unease" seem to agree, although one may search in vain for a closer definition, sometimes even described as "pain". Since this sensation is one of the root causes of obesity, if my theory is correct, a proper understanding of exactly what constitutes "hunger" is vitally important to anyone attempting to understand an obesity problem. Like thirst, hunger is a very strong sensation, although unlike thirst, its satisfaction can be deferred or even denied by the individual. There does appear to be some heritable genetic trait, particularly regarding the sequence or body priority in locating fat stores. This exists in addition to the clear influence of situational or environmental effects on caloric intake. Different storage priorities may also be sex and age related.

Beginnings of Hunger Learning

Exactly when a newborn infant learns that crying can evoke a care-taker response that will cause relief of discomfort, be it cold, hunger, or thirst is not known, but the realization must come shortly after birth. Apparently, soon after the development of thirst recognition comes the recognition of the sensation of hunger, for which there are more complex explanations. Certainly any parent who has been awakened in the middle of the night by a normal two-week-old baby can confirm that crying behavior is a very early learned way for the infant to communicate its distress. Whether this behavior is genetically controlled is moot, although it is also common throughout the animal kingdom (witness cold or hungry puppies whimpering shortly after birth). Subsequent caretaker reaction and modification of this behavior is an early imposition of socially acceptable conduct (for example: an harassed mother trying to calm her crying baby in a crowded shopping mall).

Manipulative Aspects of Hunger

That hunger can be another opportunity for manipulation seems undeniable. Too often, I have been addressed by a child with: "I'm hungry", followed quickly by the demand "FIX IT!" However, early in life food intake is learned as a behavior that tends to satisfy the hunger sensation, at least for a short while. Soon it is also recognized as a manipulative opportunity. Whether this behavior is learned before birth, shortly after, or is actually inherited in the developing individual is moot, since the inevitable result of satisfying the sensation will be by eating and its equally inevitable consequence of excess energy storage in the form of fat.

Social Aspects of Food

The social aspects of food, in both preparation and consumption, are an integral part of life and many customs have evolved around food and drink in various parts of the world, some quite elaborate and exquisite (e.g. the Japanese Tea Ceremony or English High Tea), others less formal (e.g. the American Coffee Break). Many customs have developed around agriculture as well. Although the gathering or production of foods is a time honored pursuit, from the first hunters and gatherers to the present industrial agronomist, one only has to observe the numbers of cook books available to recognize the importance of food preparation, tradition and consumption in our society.

Social Pressure to Eat

Because of human nature and societal expectations related to food ingestion, it is natural enough to find people who will respond more to others than to their own sense of the correct course for themselves. (A good example is peer pressure within adolescent groups.) The emotional support to be gained from fellow reducers has led to a huge reducing industry. The social pressures to eat derive not only from longstanding customs, but also from the fear of disease, particularly Tuberculosis (known as the White Plague or Consumption). In the past it was believed that hearty or robust appearing individuals did not harbor this dreaded infection, and therefore one could avoid at least the appearance of this devastating disease, if not actually be thwarting "consumption" itself. Revision of this societal thinking has lagged recognition of the bacterial etiology and treatment of Tuberculosis. Recent emergence of so-called "bullet-proof" (antibiotic resistant) strains of the tubercle bacillus may defeat attempts to change this apparently ingrained thinking. In addition, marked weight loss is now also associated with malignant disease, usually cancer, and a successful weight loser needs to be able to defend against friendly and well intentioned intimations of ill health, perhaps best accomplished by citing the dangers of obesity. Cancerophobia is an equivalent of tuberculophobia, and just as potentially harmful to the successful weight loss candidate.

Conditioned Responses to Food

Pavlov, the Russian physiologist, showed at the beginning of the last century by repeatedly ringing a bell before feeding, the effect on a dog's saliva flow. His experiment demonstrated that a sufficiently strong association could be established between the bell ringing and increased saliva (a digestive juice) flow that the flow eventually could be increased simply by ringing the bell, without actually feeding the dog. We can't be sure, but we can suspect that humans are subject to similar influences. If so, the rituals which tend to accumulate around food, both preparation and consumption, can be suspected to lead to a sense that food needs to be taken in. This may also operate when the eater is faced with the potential wasting of already prepared food. It is not the operant psychological thrust when an overwhelming food compulsion takes over (a basis for "food addiction," see Chapter 19 for more on this subject).

Excess Energy Storage

We have seen that the body has a tremendous capacity to chemically manipulate the food building blocks it receives through the diet. The potential energy contained within the chemical bonds in the various foods is most readily measured by counting the food's caloric value. This allows comparison between the several foods, but like a pound of feathers and a pound of lead, Calories are equal, regardless of the source. Thus, when we state that carbohydrates and proteins both yield four Calories per dry gram, we are really comparing the amounts of potential chemical energy that can be obtained from each type of carbohydrate or protein. Inherently true is the corollary that the respective breakdown or chemical unbundling of these foods will yield the same amount of energy after absorption. Since the most space-efficient way for bodies to store energy chemically is in fat (that is, on an energy per volume basis), we might expect that fat would have a higher caloric value. Indeed, this is the case as fat contains nine calories per Gram.

The body's manipulation of the chemical building blocks (amino acids and simple sugars) results in fat creation and storage, when excess energy is available. Of course, it hasn't been very long in evolutionary terms since our food supply was not all that reliable, and this storage feature is thought to have conferred a distinct survival advantage, for which we were selected by surviving. Now, the complications of overuse of the storage feature are becoming increasingly apparent.

Obsessions and Compulsions

In some cases of neurotic symptomatology, obsessions are powerful, even irresistible ideas or thoughts, while compulsions are physical acts carried out as a result of obsessive thoughts. If the thought is an irrational desire for food, the compulsive act will be eating. Of course, most obesity, although readily blamed on compulsive eating, is not actually due to satisfaction of a neurotic compulsion, although it can be. Anxiety preceding the compulsive act and the relief of anxiety from its performance can be powerful motivators. An opposite mechanism can produce anorexia.

Anxieties

Anxiety is another neurotic symptom as well as a diagnosis that may be triggered by an emotional conflict. It can result in physical signs that, although generally insubstantial, nevertheless can be bothersome and annoying. Acute anxiety can progress into a more chronic form of the disorder.

Binges

When applied to eating, Webster's definition of binge behavior as "unreserved or excessive indulgence" or "abandonment to the activity" seems to fit. Reports of Roman eating orgies, interrupted only by the need to empty a full stomach by self-induced vomiting simply to make room for more food have survived the intervening centuries and they have probably been duplicated in other cultures. More recent excessive food consumption, for whatever reason, seems much more likely to happen when the individual is alone, at any time of the day or night. And although no duration is implied in the definition, when applied to alcohol, binges can last from days to weeks, whereas when applied to food, a shorter duration is customary.

Denial

Treating denial of food consuming behaviors is a very important part of obesity management. Unfortunately, the first denial is the denial of the operation of this very mechanism. The denier is likely to report a number of primarily psychological symptoms and to ascribe those symptoms to the lack of food and the almost immediate relief of those symptoms by the ingestion of food, although we know that the digestive processes don't happen that quickly.

Water Confusion and Denial

Another refuge frequently employed by the denier or the facilitator is the assignment of excess body weight to water accumulation. Although water can and actually does contribute to total body weight, its presence is integral to a healthy state. Excess water, over the normal needs, will be excreted quickly, leaving behind only that portion needed to provide appropriate dilution of Salt (mostly KCl & NaCl) ingested and absorbed from the intestine (see Chapter 20: "Water as an Obfuscator") and that already present. Certainly on a day-to-day basis excess salt ingestion can be expected to reach a steady state, although the excess water held within the body by that salt may also contribute to blood pressure elevation. Ignorance or denial of this fact by hypertensive patients frequently causes persistence of dangerously elevated blood pressure levels with the attendant danger of Stroke. Water is not the primary offender here, but the excess Sodium is.

Dietary Recidivism (Yo-yo weight)

One of Webster's definitions of "recidivism" describes "a tendency to relapse into a previous condition" and this exactly fits the plight of an individual who has successfully struggled to reduce weight without realizing the need to change his general attitude towards or thinking about food. Unfortunately, it is widely found that 90-95% of individuals achieving significant weight loss regain a large portion of the loss, or even exceed their starting weight, when followed for a period of 3 to 5 years. Obviously, this is not only a common problem, but one which should be relatively easy to correct, given the individual's initial success. Clearly, each individual's understanding of the requirement for ongoing and life-long vigilance is a necessary and vital part of any weight control program. No associated need should exist for any further expenditure, if a successful initial control program comes after significant emotional and financial cost, but an equivalent profit motive may not exist for a good follow-up program from the successful initiators of the loss. Consequently, most weight control programs are correspondingly weak, because they lack a good follow-up program.

Part Three

Your Stomach, The Liar

Chapter 18

***Erroneous Sensations of Hunger,
Mandatory Energy Processing,
Processed Energy, Storage Locations,
Excess Energy, Losing It, How Your
Stomach Lies !***

Erroneous Sensations of Hunger

Unfortunately, neither the recency nor the quantity of food consumed give reliable indications of when, or even what, we should plan on eating again. We know that gastric wall muscle action occurs during the digestive phase while food is actually in the Stomach. However, it also occurs when the Stomach is empty. This is sometimes sensed as "growling," frequently within a few hours of a meal, whether the size of the meal was excessive or not and whether or not the Stomach is actually empty. Given that the smooth muscle of the stomach wall contracts periodically, although that organ may be empty, sensations arising from the sensory nerve endings within the stomach wall become unreliable indicators of the body's actual need, any more than the noise made when gas (probably 95% of which is swallowed air) is being audibly massaged either in the Stomach or farther down in the Intestine. Thinking that the Stomach is sending a message, when that is not the actual case, is postulated as the source of most overeaters' problems.

By paying too close attention to the signals we receive from our Stomachs telling us to eat, we tend to create an oversupply of food or potential chemical energy. It is most likely, in this way, aided by the brain's lack of understanding, that the Stomach lies.

Mandatory Energy Processing

Food taken into the body, digested, and absorbed, as indicated in the book's second section, will be stored automatically if the potential energy supplied by that food is not presently needed for body maintenance. The excess energy value will be converted automatically by the body's wonderful normal chemical processes, without any conscious input, to storage, first to a Liver glycogen, then to the more space efficient storage method of fat formation and deposition.

Fat stores are laid down throughout the body, and a little amount of fat is a very healthy resource to have available. When the immediate caloric demands or current energy needs of the body are not being met by the current food intake, or the energy or caloric balance is negative, those previously deposited fat energy stores can be drawn upon and will make up the difference, or energy deficit. It is easy to see why this trait has had a real survival advantage in earlier times, for instance, over a hard winter.

Processed Energy

When the caloric demands or current energy needs of the body are not being met by the current food intake, the energy or caloric balance is negative, and the fat energy stores will be drawn upon and will make up the difference, or energy deficit. By paying attention too closely to the signals we receive from our Stomachs telling us to eat, we tend naturally to create an oversupply of food or chemical energy to our bodies. As is the case opposite to negative energy balance, this excess energy taken in is automatically converted by the body to energy storage, although that may be contrary to our immediate, or even long-term health goals. Once the energy is stored, it will only be released when decreased intake, increased use, or both, create what amounts to a negative energy balance. However, for ongoing energy requirements, no change in the rate of energy use will result in no change in overall body weight, provided that energy intake is unchanged.

Storage Location

Much has been made of the location of excess energy stores. Supposedly, the location of fat or excess energy stores in the buttocks and thighs is associated with lower morbidity and mortality than that found in people who tend to store their excess within the abdominal cavity and in the abdominal subcutaneous tissue. Practically speaking, although the difference between the former so-called "pear shape" and the latter so-called "apple shape" probably has more to do with the apparent tendency of females to tolerate the ravages of overnutrition better than men. Men, especially overweight or obese men, tend to die at a younger age than overweight women, but the distinction seems to have little advantage.

Excess Energy

It is crucial for the overweight person to understand that potential energy in the form of food taken into the body, digested, and absorbed will be converted and stored automatically if the energy supplied by that food is not currently needed for body maintenance. The stored energy is available as an emergency energy supply. Problems develop when the first step of this emergency energy supply storage mechanism is over-used. Without willing it, the unneeded potential energy will have been converted to energy storage, perhaps contrary to our immediate, or even long-term goal. In this way unhealthily excessive stores of fat are accumulated whenever an imbalance exists between potential energy intake and energy utilization. Since the energy storage mechanism is automatic and efficient, if the energy balance remains positive, fat will be manufactured and deposited in various storage sites scattered throughout the body, and the individual's weight will increase.

Losing It

Once the potential energy is stored in body fat, it will be released only when a current undersupply of energy is created by decreased intake or increased requirement or both. But for ongoing requirements, no change in the basal rate of energy use will result in no change in overall weight, thus creating the attitude "but Doctor, I don't eat that much! (since I only eat when I'm hungry.)" When attempts to reduce weight excess are successful through a combination of increasing energy use (exercising) and lowering energy intake (dieting) each pound lost becomes the equivalent of not eating a pound of butter, ignoring the contribution of water to the overall weight. Consequently, although a little fat is not only desirable, but essential, for good health, excessive stores of fat will be accumulated inevitably whenever there exists an imbalance favoring energy intake over energy utilization.

How Your Stomach Lies

From the forgoing, it can be seen that, given normal intestinal sensation, someone who lacks access to knowledge of the basic biochemical facts of nutrition and some consequent insight into how the body handles the fuel presented to it daily by food, could easily have been mislead into thinking that a sensation of hunger was a reliable source of information. This gradually occurred to me after many frustrating discussions with patients regarding their obesity. Although there is always a danger of oversimplifying a complex subject, like nutrition, the apparent general lack of understanding of the causes of obesity makes the risk of trying to present an unbiased account of nutritional processes worth taking. It is the author's fond hope that this book will enlighten and ease the obvious job of reorienting the thinking of overweight people, It seems that a previously uninformed approach to food is causal in the development of obesity and an additional and unnecessary burden carried by overweight persons. Since even ten or twenty pounds is too much excess for some, anyone in an advanced society with its easy access to food could improve their chances for a longer and more enjoyable and productive life by developing the requisite insight that goes with a normal weight, whatever that is.

Chapter 19

*Partial-, Half- and Non-truths:
"Calories Don't Count," High Protein
Diets, Protein Sparing,
"Carbohydrates Provide Vitamins,"
High Fat Diets, "Complex"
Carbohydrates, Food Addictions,
Eating Compulsion, "Empty" Calories,
Fallacious "A Few Extra Harmless
Pounds," "Middle Aged Spread,"
Cellulite, "Normal"*

"Calories Don't Count"

"Calories Don't Count" is undoubtedly the most pernicious, outrageous, and least dependable statement that has ever been made in the area of nutritional misinformation. Although an attractive concept and title of a difficult to find book (Simon and Schuster, 1961), perhaps stated with some of the information given in previous chapters, the title is totally merit-less and misleading and will be a source of misery if relied on. In actual fact, Calories, or really kilocalories (1000 calories each), are a true measure of the potential energy stored within the inter-atomic bonds of various foods and therefore a perfectly legitimate way to make comparisons between the energy stored in, and potentially available from, various foodstuffs.

What is frequently lost sight of is the concept of the amount or dry weight of the particular food being consumed. Since neither indigestible fiber, water nor air can contribute to body energy supplies, the content of each noncaloric or unavailable component (primarily water or indigestible and therefore unab-sorbable fiber) in each food must be taken into consideration as an exception when measuring a food's true caloric value. Obviously, this becomes extremely complex when designing a lower caloric intake in a "balanced" diet. Of course, the amount of each portion is just as, if not more significant for someone limiting his or her proposed energy or caloric intake.

High Protein Diets

We have seen that as long as the needed minimal amount of each "essential" amino acid is provided, carbohydrates will be used first to provide the requisite "essential" demands of the organism for chemical energy or calories. Then, if the basic requirements for the amino acids are already met, and there is an excess of energy containing protein or amino acids available, as may happen when carbo-hydrates are restricted in some reducing diets, the nitrogen bearing molecules from the protein source will be burned to supply energy calories. A higher intake of Amino Acids in the form of proteins will result in increased Ammonia (NH_3) production. Another apparent consequence of high protein diets and carbohy-drate restriction is the production of ketones. Whether or not the ketones have delayed ill-effects is simply not known, although they are common in Diabetic coma. Any other delayed effects of the high protein diets are also unknown. That the calories derived from the proteins are more expensive to produce and acquire than those derived from carbohydrates is certain.

Protein Sparing

If even more energy or calories are taken in as food, this excess energy will be converted automatically by the body to sugars, then glycogens and ultimately stored as fat. This is an inescapable truth. Similarly, the opposite is true, that is, if available, carbohydrates are used for calories or energy, in preference to or before proteins or amino acids are burned for energy (see Chapter 19 on protein sparing). Unfortunately, the unwary can be confused or mislead by these facts being blurred or some of them being entirely omitted. When carbohydrates are burned in preference to proteins, the phenomenon is called "protein sparing". The existence of this mechanism can be a source of confusion.

"Carbohydrates Provide Vitamins"

The astute reader will already have enough information to see the error in the following: "Carbohydrates also provide vitamins-primarily B complex and vitamin C." pg48, Healthy Kids magazine, Feb/Mar'95 issue. Obviously the writer was talking about the water-soluble vitamin group as tending to be found in the same foods as the carbohydrates (see Chapter 2), but vitamins are clearly NOT carbohydrates. That particular statement appeared in an otherwise reliable magazine bearing the seal of the American Academy of Pediatrics.

The High Fat Diets

Because fats in the Stomach slow the rate of Gastric emptying and therefore the rate of digestion, the notion has been advanced that by retarding Gastric emptying with high fat feeding, there will occur a slowing down of the digestive processes and consequently less absorption of food energy. Unfortunately, although the first part about slower Gastric emptying is true, the fallacy lies in the second part. Since the digestive wheels grind exceedingly fine and, although Stomach emptying is undoubtedly retarded by the presence of fats therein, the eaten fats will ultimately be absorbed and deliver 9 Calories per gram consumed, as opposed to the 4 Calories per gram of either proteins or carbohydrates when eaten and absorbed. The theory is correct in that retarding Gastric emptying results in delayed onset of hunger sensations, but given that these sensations are unreliable anyway, the caloric/weight-loss cost/benefit ratio is prohibitively high.

Besides, the ultimate physiologic cost of prolonged ketosis, a byproduct of these diets, is unknown.

"Complex" Carbohydrates

The phrase "Complex Carbohydrates," or "Carbs" has become a watchword for people trying to lose weight and control a tendency to rely on sweets or a junk food "fix". The implication is that by taking in foods that require another digestive step, like the intestinal chemical unbundling of starches into their component sugars, time and the urge to eat more will pass. Although that may be true, the inherent fallacy here is that there is no caloric gain cost in the consumption of complex carbohydrates (as opposed to simple sugars). Therefore, so the theory goes, the reverse, or caloric gain can be avoided by the consumption of complex carbohydrates. Since the complex carbohydrates provide exactly the same caloric equivalent of the same dry weight of the simple sugars, the sole advantage of substituting chemically more complex carbohydrates apparently lies in their ever so slightly more complicated and prolonged chemical breakdown within the intestine, and consequently slightly slowed absorption.

However, if the dieter substitutes carbohydrates and fiber for fat containing snacks (e.g. raw carrots for deep fried potato chips), the caloric intake difference can be appreciable (4/9ths). And the differences between the higher fat content of most "junk" foods and either complex or simple carbohydrates is the real advantage gained when the substitution is made.

Food Addictions

A large body of literature has emerged under the rubric of "Food Addiction". The word "Addiction" has been used in association with the word "Food" to describe a clinical condition very similar to that encountered in true addictive states. The Oxford Dictionary of the English Language defines "Addiction" as being "bound to" or "devoted to," usually involving self-deliverance, apparently originally derived from Roman legal language. However, in true addiction there exists a craving, absolute need, or overwhelming desire for the addicting substance or behavior, with unpleasant withdrawal effects, particularly when deprived of the substance (not necessarily true of gambling). Moreover, the addicting substance or activity is not vital to ongoing life requirements (for instance, nicotine, alcohol, or heroin).

The vital need for almost daily food is a crucial difference between food and addicting substances or behaviors. Since some form of energy or caloric intake is absolutely necessary to the continuation of the body's metabolic or ongoing life processes on an almost daily basis, ultimately, food is just as essential as water or oxygen. Medical usage of the term "addiction" has evolved into almost exclusive reference to A) unnecessary-for-life compounds (e.g. nicotine, mood altering substances) or activities (e.g. gambling) and B) unpleasant withdrawal effects when the behavior is stopped, as well as C) the life-long process required as part of recovery. The concept of excessive habituation to the neglect of health (physical and/or financial) is implied. Nevertheless, foods can be thought of as potentially dangerous when excessively consumed, and perhaps, therefore, "addicting" is marginally appropriate. However, that usage stretches the usefulness of the word, because foods are just as necessary to continued health and life as are water or air. Therefore, use of the word "Addiction" seems misplaced, or an overbroad application of what has become a very useful medical concept. That "compulsive" food eating behaviors occur is not debatable. But applying the term "addiction" to describe behaviors which have many similar characteristics to so-called "addictive" behaviors may be desirable in educating persons who don't understand the sources of their compulsive behaviors. However, it is certainly at least an overbroad use of an otherwise well-established and very useful medical concept. That obesity is dangerous is not being protested here; indeed, the opposite. But calling overconsumption of energy or calories "addiction" is. (Ref: Katherine, A., "Anatomy of a Food Addiction", Prentice Hall/Parkside 1991, e.g. "Habituation to food means depending psychologically on food" and "Physical dependence" equals "Physical addiction".)

"Eating Compulsion"

Understanding the underlying driving force behind excessive food consumption can lead into many unexplored mental channels. It may be hoped that deeper psychological insights will have an additive effect to the information being provided in this book.

"Empty" Calories

As we have seen, vitamins are special kinds of food without caloric or energy supplying value, but necessary for normal body functions. Energy (AKA calories) can be supplied by various foods and most foods contain some vitamins. The concept of "Empty Calories" has arisen from more or less pure foods that do not contain any of the essentials (e.g. vitamins or amino acids). However the attractive notion is that if the Calories are "empty," they have no caloric impact. Therefore, they don't add to the total energy consumed. This is simply false. If there are available calories present in the food, and they are consumed, they will be digested and absorbed.

Fallacious "A Few Extra Harmless Pounds"

There seems to be a widespread belief that post-adolescents can accumulate "a few extra harmless pounds" beyond their teen years (ignoring the serious implications of childhood obesity), without incurring any ultimate life-shortening price. Although the evidence to counter that thought would require a long-term study, which has yet to be financed or done, the contrary makes eminent common sense. By reviewing the table in Figure 7.5, it should be apparent that any post adolescence gain in weight can have very few sources in a supposedly "healthy" adult. If energy, or fat, is stored in all the common sites, a small fraction of that storage must take place in vulnerable arterial walls, thereby laying the groundwork for later strokes or heart attacks. Since fat is so easy to accumulate, and so hard to lose, it makes sense to try to avoid the accumulation, in the first place.

"Middle Aged" Spread

Just as we lack a definition for an "old" human, we have no absolute point at which we can say middle age starts. Generally speaking, 30 years after birth seems about right, although thirty-somethings might object to middle age starting at 30 and ending at 60. Some might prefer that middle age be defined as starting at 40, particularly those in the affected decade. Then, if we were to consider that middle age lasts 30 years, it would extend to 70 before old age sets in, but somehow that seems too old for "middle" age. In any case, a common observation, remarked in the concept of "middle age spread" is that aging beyond young adulthood is accompanied by the accumulation of fat in both sexes, particularly in more affluent societies. No general agreement exists as to the cause of this phenomenon, be it declining exertion or energy use in the middle years, metabolic slowdown, or relative or absolute increased energy intake, or a combination of these factors. Women who survive their reproductive function, and most now do, on the average outlive men of similar age by almost ten years. Whether this is due to the internal hormone environment of females, to external factors, or to some unknown combination of causes has never been worked out. The observation has been made that heavy older women tend to deposit their excess energy stores in the lower lumbar regions, buttocks, and thighs. Attempts have been made to compare the relative size of these so-called "pear" shaped deposits with the primarily abdominal deposits so common in middle aged men, the so-called "apple" shape, and to connect the difference in mortality, in particular cardiac mortality, to this distribution difference. Unknown is the mortality difference between "pear shaped" men and "apple shaped" men, although that might finally determine the question, were it possible to isolate it. Clearly, neither accumulation can be considered "healthy".

Cellulite

The second college edition of the American Heritage Dictionary defines the word "cellulite" as "A fatty deposit, as around the thighs and buttocks". However, the final arbiter of the English language, the Oxford Standard Dictionary, does not yet even recognize the existence of the word or problem. Cellulite does seem to exist and to be associated with unsightly skin wrinkling, probably due to the stretched fibrous attachments of skin to the underlying fascia with former excessive fatty deposits in the intervening subcutaneous fat cells. One might even conjecture that the process of laying down "cellulite", with the associated stretching of those subcutaneous fibrous attachments might play an etiologic role in the development of "stretch marks," for instance during pregnancy or obesity, with some subsequent weight loss.

Much seems to be made of the existence of "cellulite," particularly in periodicals mostly aimed at the feminine half of the younger generation, offering, for most part, beauty tips. There are even vacuum massagers for sale which are described as having "skin smoothing" capabilities. Since the "cellulite" appearance is most likely originally due to stuffed fat cells within a limited subcutaneous space, bounded by multiple fibrous bands binding the muscle surrounding deep fascia to the underside of the overlying skin, or dermis, it would seem that the best way to avoid "cellulite" is to avoid overstuffing those subcutaneous fat cells. This tendency may also be responsible for the production of "stretch marks" in the skin by the scarring produced within the stretched subcutaneous fibrous bands, made more visible after weight loss.

"Normal"

What's to be considered normal? Unfortunately, no good standard exists. The only reference source is the age, height, and weight tables for men and women from the Life insurers that tend to reflect the present overfed state of the adult American population (those applying for Life Insurance). If our fullback were included at age 40, even at his lower weight there would be a much larger percentage of fat (and, presumably, hard arteries) represented in the tables, as many suspect. On the other hand, the relationship between excess weight and complications due to hard arteries and other problems (e.g. development of Diabetes, Pulmonary Emboli, or higher Surgical mortality) has been repeatedly demonstrated and is undeniable.

Chapter 20

Sodium, Water, Calculating Intake, Water Weight Obfuscation, When to Weigh, Ideal Body Weight, PMS

Sodium

The element Sodium (symbol Na, as in NaCl, Sodium Chloride, or Table Salt) can be responsible for water retention in addition to many other problems. Sodium tends to be kept outside the cells. If, for one reason or another, an individual cannot maintain a balanced low level of total body sodium, there will be an almost automatic (so-called obligatory) retention of water. As the body tries to dilute the retained salt, sodium and water tend first to accumulate in all the extracellular spaces including the blood serum. Although the greater amount of total body water is intracellular (about 2/3 intracellular; about 1/3 extracellular), if the water the sodium causes to be held within the body is excessive, it increases total extracellular volume. In this case, total body fluid (particularly blood volume) increases above normal. The excess fluid accumulates in all the extracellular spaces, starting with the lowest and responding to the force of gravity first. Consequently, feet or ankles tend to swell before other parts. If one lower extremity has been damaged previously, that member will be more prone to swelling before its partner.

Once again, the body can be tricked into behaving as though the sodium level were not really high, and the kidneys can be fooled with medication into excreting potassium, which will draw out water with it. This is the basis for the use of several "water pills" to lose weight but, as with thyroid hormone, the cost/ultimate benefit ratio is too high for weight control. And the effect will disappear when the unneeded medication is stopped, as it should never have been started in the first place.

It is this tendency to accumulate fluid and cause an increase in the blood volume that has lead to the recommendation for people with weak hearts or high blood pressure to lower their level of salt consumption, and consequently reduce their blood volume. The extra heart effort needed to circulate the expanded blood is thereby reduced.

Water

Since water itself has no nutritional or caloric value, it is one of the very few substances that can be consumed without any negative long-term weight consequences. The other non-calorics are indigestible fiber (celluloses), and air which is 20% oxygen. We already understand why water is such a significant part of ongoing cell life processes. If water were weightless, we would have no difficulty understanding that any completely absorbable particular food's energy content would be directly related to its weight (like the dry weight) of that particular food. Unfortunately that is not the case. The calorically inert (both water and fiber percentage) of each food must be allowed for and entered into any calculation of that particular food's nutritional, or "Caloric" value.

Calculating Intake

For example, in deriving, an estimate of Calories to be consumed, if one were preparing wheat cereal or oatmeal porridge for breakfast, one needs to know the water and indigestible fiber content of the prepared cereal to gain true insight into the amount of nutrition being consumed. The weight of the cooked cereal not only depends on it's ultimate water content, that is, how much water was used originally, but how much boiled off during cooking, and how much was absorbed by the grain. Also the amount of water in the milk added after cooking needs to be considered. Although everyone seems to understand that watery, or highly diluted, porridge is not very nutritious, the noncaloric part of the cereal is very difficult to determine.

Similarly, the amount of water and fiber contained in such a simple fruit as a grape has no caloric effect. The sugar content and the minimal protein content actually represent a small portion of the grape's weight, but they represent all of the grape's nutritional content. Since most fruits also contain indigestible fiber, this can add to any fruit's weight without changing its caloric value. Although the fiber has no caloric effect, there may be other benefits from consumption of that fiber.

Milk is another source of potential confusion. The Federally mandated nutritional percentage container labels on milk refer only to the actual butterfat (9 Calories per gram) content, e.g. 2% means 2 grams Butterfat in 100 grams of milk. However, the greater part of the milk is water and that part is calorically neutral. On the other hand, the milk sugar and digestible protein in the milk are both food and can be relied on to provide 4 Calories per gram each. Also, the fat (butterfat) in the milk is now treated (homogenized) in order to remain suspended throughout the water, whereas before the homogenization treatment it would rise to the top as cream. By adding homogenized milk and perhaps a little sugar and fruit to the cereal, one is actually creating a very complex mixture of nutrients, or life-giving chemicals, for one's simple breakfast. The nutritional story becomes increasingly complex throughout the day.

Water Weight Obfuscation

The assignment of excess body weight to water accumulation is sometimes valid, although frequently not. Although water can and actually does contribute to total body weight, its presence is absolutely necessary for a healthy state. However, since excess water, over normal requirements, is quickly excreted, it only leaves behind that portion required to provide appropriate dilution of salts (mostly KCl and NaCl) ingested and absorbed from the intestine. In addition, that water already present within the food or that derived from metabolism or the burning of the food becomes a part of the total body water intake. Usually, on a day-to-day basis, if an excess of salt is ingested, the body level can be expected to reach a plateau. However, the excess water retained within the body by the excess Sodium Chloride can contribute to falsely high weight and blood pressure elevation, as well. Water is not the primary offender here, but Sodium is.

When to Weigh

In following one's weight pattern from day-to-day, it is prudent to determine comparable levels. In order to do this, a convenient time and body status must be chosen and adhered to, since there can be wide variations throughout the day particularly in bowel and bladder content. Of course, clothing status also participates in weight. The most opportune time of day is usually just after bowel and bladder evacuation, after awaking, and similarly dressed, from day to day (i.e. shoes, slippers, or barefoot). Although frequently maladjusted, undisturbed scales usually give reliable measurements that are comparable on a day-to-day basis, but not necessarily comparable between different scales.

Ideal Body Weight

What is the ideal weight? As is so often the case when facts are not well established, arguments justifying one position or another may be made, ad infinitum, with no or little regard for the truth, essentially because the truth is unknown. Unfortunately, this is the case with respect to "ideal" or "best" body weight.

In addition to the infinite individual variety we accept and prefer as normal, we acknowledge and accept the individual differences between sexes, skin pigmentation, hair growth, physical ability, and intelligence. There also seems to be ready agreement, among those willing to face the truth, that pain should be avoided, that infectious processes should be controlled and their effects minimized. Also that, where possible, degenerative diseases should be controlled, and that cancers or other forms of new growths should be avoided, or, at least, diagnosed and treated early, and that, in avoidance, known environmental carcinogen exposure should be minimized. We agree that aging and death are inevitable, although not necessarily related, the latter to be postponed as long as possible. In none of these areas of common agreement, except the last, does weight appear to be a factor.

However, we do know that blockages tend to build up within aging arteries, particularly those supplying vital organs like the heart and brain. Also we know that the incidence of heart attacks and strokes has increased, particularly in ours and other more affluent societies, where the earlier scourges have been controlled, if not eliminated. We know that those blockages begin with fatty deposits, mostly cholesterol, in aging arteries. Our knowledge does not firmly extend into the relationship between excessive weight and the apparent increasing incidence of vascular and other problems, although it does make good common sense to see a possible relationship.

Admitting that a definitive answer cannot be given to the question "What is the best weight for me?," one is lead to speculate that the closest approximation to what might prove to be the ultimately correct response is five or ten percent more than your best weight when you were a young adult. What shape were you in then? Had you been active? Did you take part in any sports? Were you ever in excellent physical condition? If yes, what was you're weight then? Assuming that most skeletal and muscle growth occurs before early adulthood, the weight of early adulthood is the one we should probably seek (since any subsequent addition would be due to fat accumulation, ignoring the weight of replaced muscle). This assumption relies on the absence of childhood obesity. Referring again to the subsection on density in Chapter 8, the body's behavior in a swimming pool can give a quick and reasonably accurate indication of the amount of fat present in any individual. If the buoyancy of the body, even with the lungs full of air, is negative (that is, one tends to sink), then one's total specific gravity is greater than 1.0. Contrariwise, if one tends to float, the body's fat is supplying the buoyancy, in addition to the buoyancy supplied by the air in the respiratory and intestinal tracts. No one really knows whether a specific gravity of 1.0 is desirable, but it does provide a readily available and reasonably accurate index of the amount of body fat present. While a recommendation for major weight loss tends to be rejected advice, certainly unpopular, we all must admit that, once our skeletons get to their adult size, and our muscles achieve "normal" development, anything extra has to be fat, even if we don't believe it or show it.

PMS

Although observing and recording daily weights usually provide an excellent index of progress in weight loss or the opposite, they can be misleading, particularly in cycling women, or in people who retain Sodium or Table Salt (NaCl) and water, usually because of heart failure. The onset of the menstruation cycle is a clear point from which to measure or begin observations, but the retained body water that is associated with the body's preparation for the onset of menstruation is released over the next day or two.

Thus, a truer index of a cycling woman's weight is more likely to be obtained when comparing weights from month to month on Day +2 or later of each cycle. The body's preparation for the monthly onset of menstruation has been associated not only with a failure of attempted weight loss or actual weight gain from retained water, but a constellation of symptoms which has come to be known as

PMS or "pre-menstrual syndrome". In addition to the electrolyte and water changes, PMS is likely due to the exceedingly complex series of internal hormonal changes that accompany the preparation of the uterus and its lining for supporting a pregnancy. Following the onset of each normal menstrual period there is a remarkable increase in the amount of urine produced by the kidneys and excreted, and a corresponding weight loss. Whether the premenstrual fluid accumulation is the cause of the PMS, or whether it is coincidental, like the occasional severe headache or the symptoms of endometriosis accompanying period onset, is moot. That it does occur and demands consideration is the more important point.

Naturally, if one has been successfully paring down one's true weight by not ingesting and storing more energy than one is using on a daily or weekly basis, and one is subject to this inevitable accumulation of water toward the time of period onset, the actual weight measured at period onset will be a combination of the individual's true weight plus the excess water retained and, as the premenstrual water accumulation and weight rise, it is likely to be most discouraging. Therefore it makes good sense for a cycling woman to make intermonthly comparisons by using a relatively dry period, usually beyond the second day of the cycle. Pregnancy, with its marked accompanying hormonal changes, makes weight tracking even more difficult.

Chapter 21

Who or What Can You Trust?, Quantity Counts, Essentials Are, "Sustain", Food Labels, Do the Math (Chocolate Pretzels), "Loaded" Foods

The whole idea of this book is to supply reliable and unbiased information, particularly for those hoping to cope with overnourishment. Clearly "Nutrition" is a huge subject and obviously more complicated than we present, but probably as much as a result of its complexity as any volitional attempt to mislead, areas of the subject become the focus of what turn out to be misleading or incomplete thoughts or statements. So, what can be trusted?

We have seen that there are innumerable ways to confuse the willing, but inadequately informed, individual attempting to lose weight. One of the sources of confusion is in definitions. For instance, the term "carbohydrates," although meaningful by itself, has been misused to indicate sources of carbohydrates as well as the chemicals discussed in Chapter 2. By ignoring well established facts, others dwell on little more than conjecture to advocate one or another substance as "the answer" to overweight; for instance "Carbs".

Actually, much of what has been written about losing weight rings true, particularly the lists of caloric values of various foods. For the most part, these schedules are reliable.

Quantity Counts

What is less frequently noted is the great variety of "amount." One needs only to consider the size of one potato available in most markets, varying perhaps from about 30 grams to over 200 grams, to realize the difficulty in measuring one potato's caloric value. Water content of each potato also can vary considerably, both before and after cooking. Further complicating the picture is the problem of how much fat-containing butter or other lipid, as well as what type of fat (i.e. absorbable and therefore calorie bearing or not), might be added in the preparation of the potato (for instance in frying or deep fat frying), how much water or indigestible fiber is contained in the ultimate food, and whether anything will interfere with the digestive, absorptive, or utilization processes. Thus, a series of uncertainties ensues.

Essentials Are Just That

What is true is that all the "essential" needs must be met, including all the various substances mentioned as essential earlier. Although some of the requirements are only now being demonstrated by their absence from defined intravenous feedings or "elemental" diets, administered via the intestine, some of the requirements are well understood and none may be ignored. Most of the less well defined requirements are needed in such tiny amounts that the average eater will take in the needed amount as food contaminants. This seems to be particularly true for the small amounts of needed minerals.

We are left with many uncertainties. This is simply reflective of the incompleteness of the present state of our knowledge. However, most of the information given here is generally well accepted and designed to provide insight, albeit admittedly and necessarily incomplete, into the intimate nutritional workings of our bodies. Most of the more prominent medical journal editors and the U. S. Federal Health authorities seem to be aware of the huge information deficit problem facing our society in the next century The editors are trying to select contributions to their journals that will add to the public's knowledge and the ability of the overweight afflicted to cope with their problem. "The aim of weight reduction should be to decrease morbidity rather than to meet a cosmetic standard of thinness, and obese persons should be encouraged to set reasonable short-term goals for weight loss, bearing this in mind. They must recognize that any lifestyle alterations, in the form of increased exercise or decreased caloric intake (*or both*), made to lose weight will need to be continued indefinitely." From an article by M. Rosenbaum, et al. "Medical Progress: Obesity" New England Journal of Medicine v377: pp 402-3, 1997.

"Sustain"

Several other authors have used the word "sustain", and this seems to be the crux of the weight losing matter. Unfortunately, there is no way to increase one's caloric intake and to lose weight in the process. Nor is there any magic pill. Although some substances and items will cause temporary imbalance (for instance the tendency of oily foods to inhibit Stomach contractions, supposedly thereby limiting hunger sensations), the ultimate result can either be that the lipid is digested and absorbed (and utilized or stored) at 9 Cal/gram or it is not digested or absorbed and causes diarrhea. It may be apocryphal, but there is an old story of a wonderful diet pill that worked very well. Later it was discovered that these wonderful pills contained tapeworm eggs, and the pleased successful dieters were feeding their new worms as well as themselves. Needless to say, the Food and Drug Administration would never have approved, had it been in existence when those pills were marketed. Thankfully, so severe a treatment is no longer available.

Food Labels

The Federal required food labels are very helpful in calculating one's actual intake. However, caution must be exercised in comparing the amount of each nutriment in what is described as a "serving". Generally speaking, the labeled "servings" are minimal, thus one tends to take in a larger amount than described in the label, although the contents described on the label tend to be truthful and reliable for the small amounts indicated (see below). Additives, like milk to cereal, need to be calculated separately, since the ultimate caloric value will vary depending on the type and amount of additive used.

Do The Math

As an example, the Nutrition Label on a box of "typical" chocolate covered pretzels contains the following information: Serving Size: Two Pretzels (only), everything else is calculated from this small number, but, of course, the number of "servings" is between the consumer and his or her conscience. For a complete understanding of the threat each little 'goodie' represents, the calculation from these labels can be extended to any food bearing a government approved nutrition label. For instance, on the Chocolate Pretzel Box:

SERVING SIZE: (only) Two Pretzels

SUBSTANCE	Amount/Serving:	@CAL/Gm	TOTAL CAL/Serving
FATS:	Total: 5 Grams (from 2 pretzels)	x9	45
	Saturated: 4 Grams (included in the above number)		(36)
CARBOHYDRATES:	Total: 20 Grams	x4	80
	Sugar: 10 Grams (included in the 20)		(40)
PROTEINS:	Total: 2 Grams	x4	8

Total Calories from two (tiny) chocolate pretzels: <u>133</u>

(The label actually says <u>130</u>, but that probably includes some rounding downwards.)

Figure 21.1 Example of Chocolate Pretzel Box Label

Remember, the %DV, or percent daily value, has very little to do with the real, or calculated, intake. So if you consumed four of those little pretzels, you would actually have eaten 266 Calories in that short time, or with "about" 28 servings per bag, at least 130 (their number), or 133 (my number) times 28, or a total of 3724 Calories from one bag. Go figure.

"Loaded" Foods

All too frequently we hear that this vegetable or that fruit contains "loads" of this or that vitamin or mineral. In point of fact, hardly any of the various natural vitamin sources contain nearly as much as one small complete multivitamin pill. Since there is supposedly no scrambling or obscuring of information tolerated for the labeling of vitamin pills, usually the least expensive complete pill is the one to take (but note "Consumer Reports" article "Multivitamins-What to avoid, how to choose" pages 19 & 20, February 2006). Also, the way the digestive and storage processes work, vitamins need be taken only once or twice a week if the person is not on a very restricted diet. Storage of the water soluble vitamins is less certain and complete than storage of the various fat soluble vitamins, so that were one to have to find a pill source for both vitamin solubility classes, probably one pill every two weeks would be an adequate frequency for the fat soluble group. A shorter period would likely be adequate for the water solubles. Since both groups are in most multivitamin pills, as long as we present the needed chemical configuration (vitamin) to the normal digestive system fairly often, the body, in its wisdom, will take what it needs and let the unneeded pass. The final conclusion is that food labels must be reliable, that amounts of digestible and absorbable foods are important, that calories count, and that the scales don't lie. Unfortunately, the other message from the Stomach, or "feed us," as we have postulated, is totally unreliable.

About the Author

After completing training in General Surgery in Albany, NY, where, with a team, he performed the first Liver transplants, and Board Certification, Dr. Goodrich practiced for many years in Santa Fe, NM, where he first became interested in the obesity problem. Subsequently, for health reasons, he moved to the Philadelphia area where he continues a consulting practice.

Topic Index
(**Bold** Refers to Chapter Numbers)

Chapter Start Page List

978-0-595-40407-0
0-595-40407-3